Instructions for Geriatric Patients

Third Edition

 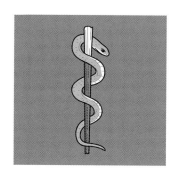 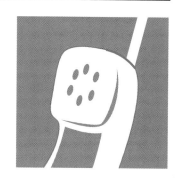

Instructions for Geriatric Patients

William A. Sodeman, Jr., M.D., J.D., F.A.C.P., F.A.C.G., F.A.C.L.M.

Professor Emeritus
Department of Medicine
Medical University of Ohio
Lecturer in Law
University of Toledo
College of Law
Toledo, Ohio

Thomas C. Sodeman, M.D.

Assistant Professor, Department of Medicine
University of South Florida
College of Medicine
Tampa, Florida

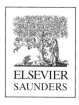

ELSEVIER
SAUNDERS

ELSEVIER
SAUNDERS
An Imprint of Elsevier

The Curtis Center
170 S Independence Mall W 300E
Philadelphia, Pennsylvania 19106

Instructions for Geriatric Patients, ed 3 ISBN: 1-4160-0203-0

NOTICE

Medicine is an ever-changing field. Standard safety precautions must be followed, but as new research and clinical experience broaden our knowledge, changes in treatment and drug therapy may become necessary or appropriate. Readers are advised to check the most current product information provided by the manufacturer of each drug to be administered to verify the recommended dose, the method and duration of administration, and contraindications. It is the responsibility of the treating physician relying on experience and knowledge of the patient, to determine dosages and the best treatment for each individual patient. Neither the Publisher nor the editor assumes any liability for any injury and/or damage to persons or property arising from this publication.

Previous editions copyrighted 1999, 1995.

Library of Congress Cataloging-in-Publication Data
Sodeman, William A. (William Anthony), 1936–
 Instructions for geriatric patients / William A. Sodeman, Thomas C. Sodeman.–3rd ed.
  p. ; cm.
 ISBN 1-4160-0203-0
 1. Geriatrics. 2. Patient education. I. Sodeman, Thomas C. II. Title.
 [DNLM: 1. Geriatrics. 2. Caregivers–psychology. 3. Patient Education. WT 100 S679i 2005]
 RC952.5.S656 2005
 618.97–dc22   2004051301

Acquisitions Editor: Daniel Pepper
Developmental Editor: Dennis DiClaudio
Publishing Services Manager: Joan Sinclair
Project Manager: Mary B. Stermel
Marketing Manager: Laura Meisky

Printed in the United States of America

Last digit is the print number: 9 8 7 6 5 4 3 2 1

For Our Wives

"A WORD IS NOT A CRYSTAL,
TRANSPARENT AND UNCHANGED,
IT IS THE SKIN OF A LIVING THOUGHT
AND MAY VARY GREATLY IN COLOR AND CONTENT
ACCORDING TO THE CIRCUMSTANCES
AND THE TIME IN WHICH IT IS USED."

———————————

Oliver Wendell Holmess, Jr., Towne V Eisner 245 U.S. 418, 425 (1918).

Preface to the Third Edition

Many studies have shown that patients only retain a fragment of what their physician tells them during face-to-face encounters. There are many reasons. These may include short visits, large amounts of technical material, or the fact that some are not auditory learners. This volume, now in its third edition, is intended to serve as a bridge between the doctor's office and the patient's home, in a sense lengthening the office visit.

The material has undergone revision and addition to reflect the changes in knowledge and revision of standards of care. We have tried to limit the technical jargon and to convey ideas clearly to those not in the medical field.

We would like to express our gratitude to our families for allowing us to take the time away from them to produce this book, and to our editors at W.B. Saunders. Finally, we would like to express our gratitude to our patients, from whom we learn at each visit, no matter how brief.

William A. Sodeman, Jr., M.D., J.D.
Thomas C. Sodeman, M.D.

Preface to the First Edition

Most physicians spend a working lifetime in conversation with patients. Much of this conversation time is spent taking a history, but equally important is the time spent on instruction about treatment. Not so long ago patients were comfortable being told what to do. They eschewed explanations about how and why their illness occurred as though illness was as mysterious as the Latin writing in the prescription. With time, the sophistication of patients has increased. Television, both programming and advertising, now supplies a vocabulary of medical terms; however, television usage might not be medically accurate, and patients often have their own unique meanings for these terms. Complexity of treatment has also increased. The opportunities for confused communication between patient and physician burgeon. Apparently not only the Shadow, but also physicians have the ability to cloud men's minds.

My goal with Instructions for Geriatric Patients is to provide simple, direct aids to patient communication. Written instructions that patients can take with them are a ready reference when confusion arises. Ambiguity, alas, is inherent in any set of instructions. No one can write a set of instructions that will meet the needs of every practice. Practice styles differ, opinions about treatment programs differ, and the emphasis given to various aspects of treatment programs differs from physician to physician. For this reason I have attempted to keep the instructions generic. It may not be easier, but it is more effective in patient management to add to the instruction sheets as you give them to the patient.

I am indebted to my wife, Marjorie C. Sodeman, who patiently read through each instruction, chiding me when I wandered from simple, direct statements into the pseudoscientific jargon that plagues much of our interaction with patients. I am equally indebted to my editors at W.B. Saunders Company for their patience and concern that the instructions remain simple and as unambiguous as possible.

I welcome comments from readers and users, corrections and recommendations for additions to the book. Instructions for Geriatric Patients will never be so encyclopedic as to be complete, but there was no intent to leave out an important problem.

William A. Sodeman, Jr., M.D.
Toledo, Ohio

Contents

9   *Cardiovascular Problems*   *181*

CHAPTER 1

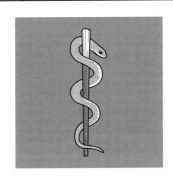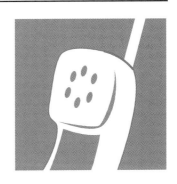

Confusion

Depression

Patient and Caregiver's Guide

General Information

Depression is a disorder of mood. Depression may vary from a mild, expected (normal) response to the stresses of daily living to a severe psychiatric disturbance that can interfere with daily living. Severe depression is often reversible and should be treated. The occurrence of depression is more frequent with aging. It is more likely to occur in people who have had a prior episode of depression or if there is a family history of depression. Physical illness, particularly chronic illness, is also a predisposing factor. Social factors, such as isolation, financial losses, and bereavement, can lead to depression as well. Losses, whether primarily physical (such as of income or a home) or emotional (such as of a spouse, a friend, or even a pet), are part of the aging process. When symptoms of depression persist for 2 or more months, a severe depression often called a *major depressive episode* is diagnosed.

Many manifestations of depression in older individuals overlap changes related to aging or changes due to other diseases. One must be careful to not overinterpret these clues. In the older patient, it is also possible for depression to present with primarily physical symptoms rather than changes in mood. This is *masked depression* and may be difficult to appreciate and difficult for the caregiver or the patient's physician to identify. Common manifestations include nervousness, insomnia, memory loss, and dizziness, all problems easily ascribed to other aging-related problems. Careful evaluation by a physician is necessary to separate depression from other causes of confusion.

Important Points in Treatment

When the patient's physician can identify a likely specific underlying cause for the depression, the therapy focuses on treating this underlying condition. Even in these cases, the patient's

3

physician may recommend supportive care by a counselor, social worker, psychologist, or psychiatrist. Supportive care of this sort can hasten recovery.

Patients with hearing and/or visual limitations often require additional help to remain integrated and active within the family and community. Isolation caused by failing special senses, sight, and hearing often aggravates depression.

Medications

Major depression with impairment of function, as well as depression without an identifiable and treatable underlying cause, may respond to the use of drug treatment. Several drugs are effective, and the most commonly used are *tricyclic anti-depressants*. These are potent medicines that have side effects. Selection of the most appropriate drug is often based on the ability to tolerate possible side effects. Careful control of the dose and the time of administration is essential to the proper and effective use of the drugs and to the management of side effects. Special attention by the caregiver is important for successful treatment.

Side effects of these medications may include, but are not limited to, dry mouth, blurred vision, urinary retention, rapid heart rate, persistent heartburn, and glaucoma attacks. Some patients may experience dizziness when they stand up. Occasionally, these drugs produce confusion, sleepiness, or bizarre or inappropriate behavior. Any abrupt behavior changes in a patient receiving drug therapy for depression should be brought to the physician's attention immediately.

The medications used for the treatment of depression are also useful in treating and managing other diseases. They are, for instance, commonly employed in the management of irritable bowel syndrome and other functional gastrointestinal complaints. Treatment with what are called "antidepressants" does not always imply the presence of depression.

Depression may also be related to substance abuse. Abuse of alcohol or illegal drugs may be a factor. Stopping the substance abuse is an important but difficult step in treatment. Seasonal depression is a feature associated with winter in northern climates. A variety of treatments with daily exposure to bright lights is helpful in alleviating this form of depression.

Notify Our Office If

- You note any clue or suggestion that the patient may have suicidal thoughts. This should be taken seriously and promptly reported to the patient's physician. Suicide is an unfortunate and not uncommon accompaniment of severe depression. The patient is often indirectly asking for help.
- Side effects of drug treatment occur. Side effects often require prompt, even immediate, intervention. These particularly include glaucoma attacks (sudden, acute pain in the eye), which may lead to blindness if not promptly treated; urinary retention, which may lead to bladder infection and damage to the kidneys; and abnormal heart rhythm, which often manifests as dizziness and, if untreated, may lead to sudden death.

Dementia

Patient and Caregiver's Guide

General Information

Dementia is a disorder of the brain. It involves the loss of memory and other mental functions. It can result from many different causes and can vary in its severity from patient to patient. Many people are familiar with Alzheimer's disease only, a degenerative dementia that accounts for half of the cases, and they are unaware of other treatable causes of dementia. Even in cases in which the underlying cause may not be readily treatable, careful management can support and extend the quality of life for the patient, family, and friends.

Dementia may include the following:
- Loss of memory, particularly recent memory
- Impairment of intellectual functions severe enough to interfere with a person's job, social life, or both
- Change in personality
- Behavioral changes, such as delusion, hallucination, or depression
- Impairment of judgment.

Generally there is an organic cause for dementia, but, in many patients, this can be difficult to identify. There is usually no impairment of consciousness. The affected person remains alert. Most dementia is progressive, but the speed of progression may be highly variable from person to person. Often it is very slow.

Evaluation by a physician is important to uncover the reversible components of the patient's dementia. In addition, every effort should be made to help the patient achieve optimal physical health. The added burden of poorly controlled high blood pressure, diabetes, or other chronic diseases may worsen the difficulties related to dementia.

Important Points in Treatment

The goal of treatment is to provide a satisfactory quality of life for the patient and caregiver. Variation in patients and in resources available to deal with individual patient's problems prevents making strict rules.

1. Encourage physical activity. Respect the patient's physical limits, but remember that lack of activity and exercise can be as detrimental to the quality of life as too much activity or exercise. Each increment of loss of fitness due to neglect of exercise has a negative effect on the patient's ability to maintain the activities of daily living.

2. Encourage good nutrition. Often this becomes a balancing act between adequate nutrition and optimal nutrition. Carefully structured diets are good only to the extent that they are eaten. The patient will eventually require help with eating.

3. Help the patient with insomnia to maintain a normal relationship with the environment. Bright lights during the day and avoidance of naps are helpful. The body has a normal day/night rhythm that needs to be reinforced.

4. Avoid challenging the limits of intellectual ability. Stick to tasks that are within the current intellectual capabilities of the patient. To maintain the current level of intellectual function, the individual must use these capabilities. Do not isolate the patient from activities of daily living. Attempt to motivate participation in everyday activities, but remember the patient's limits. Careful use of memory aids and routines can help even intellectually impaired patients remain active in daily affairs.

5. Manage the patient's environment to avoid confrontation and frustration. Simplify activities; use memory aids and safety engineering. Adjust the surroundings for ease of getting around. Encourage the use of lights.

6. Identify complications and potential complications in the management of daily living. Particularly important complications are wandering, incontinence, depression, agitation, and aggressiveness.

7. Regularly participate in the reevaluation of the patient's general health. Effective management requires changes as the dementia progresses.

8. Seek help from social services to identify community resources appropriate for the patient's level of need.

9. Seek counseling to help with legal, social, and ethical decisions regarding management choices.

10. Patients with visual and/or hearing impairment often require additional support to remain active and integrated into family and community functions.

Medications

Many of the problems associated with dementia, such as delusion, insomnia, agitation, or depression, are treatable with medication. Careful evaluation by your physician is essential to select the most appropriate drug.

Few drugs are directly useful for the management of dementia, but several new drugs are available to help slow the progression of dementia. These include tacrine (Cognex), ergoloid mesylates (Hydergine), donepezil (Aricept), rivastigmine, and galantamine. Tacrine does not reverse changes in memory function that are already present, but it does slow the progression of these changes. Therefore, it is useful as a long-term addition in the care of patients with senile dementia.

Tacrine should be taken on an empty stomach. It takes several weeks or more for a full effect. It does not seem to benefit all patients. Often there must be a trial period to see whether it will be effective for a given patient. The drug has significant side effects. These include alteration of the effects of other drugs and the possibility of some injury to the liver. Donepezil is a new drug that is similar to tacrine in its effects.

Ergoloid mesylate may provide slight improvement in thinking, but it is helpful in only a few patients. Selection of patients to receive any of these drugs requires discussion between the caregiver and the patient's physician.

Rivastigmine should be given with food to offset stomach upset with nausea, which is a common side effect. Galantamine can be taken with meals twice per day.

All of these medications are most effective in people with mild to moderate dementia. A trial period is usually required to see whether they will be effective and useful for any individual.

Many drugs that are properly given for coincident but unrelated conditions can worsen dementia or complicate its management. A careful written medication history available to all physicians involved in the patient's care, including all drugs (prescription and nonprescription), is the best defense against medication-induced complications.

Notify Our Office If

- There is any suspicion of infection or injury. Patients with impaired mentation are susceptible to infection and injury without manifesting the usual or expected complaints.
- A patient taking tacrine or donepezil complains of nausea, headache, or sore muscles.
- A patient taking tacrine or donepezil has vomiting, diarrhea, or difficulty keeping balance.
- Abrupt changes in mental status occur. Many other diseases do not necessarily present with typical symptoms, but most will produce some change in status, particularly mental status.

Delirium

Patient and Caregiver's Guide

General Information

Delirium is one of several causes of confusion. It is particularly common in elderly patients. Delirium causes the mind to become clouded. Impaired awareness of the surrounding environment occurs. This may be as minor as simple misinterpretations and inattention or as severe as frank hallucinations. Patients often seem confused or disoriented with regard to time or place and may have visual or auditory hallucinations. Memory may be impaired. Sleep is often disturbed. Delirium develops quickly, typically within hours to days. Its severity usually fluctuates throughout the day. It is easy to be fooled into thinking that the delirium has subsided only to have it reappear after an interval. Generally, there is an identifiable cause.

Delirium commonly occurs as a reaction to infections, metabolic disorders, poor heart function, small strokes, temperature imbalance, drug reactions, and even urinary or fecal retention. Environmental changes as innocent as moving a patient to new and unfamiliar surroundings, such as a nursing home, can be the cause of delirium.

Careful examination by the patient's physician is important to uncover health problems that may underlie the development of the delirium. Because delirium is associated with a wide variety of medications, it is important to make available to the physician a complete list of drugs—both prescription and nonprescription—that the patient is taking. Treatment of any underlying problem is the best way to reverse the delirious state. With proper management, the delirium usually clears in a few days, but, in a few cases, it may persist for several weeks before responding to treatment.

Important Points in Treatment

The treatment prescribed by the patient's physician for underlying conditions is of primary importance. Measures that focus mostly on the patient's environment are equally important in speeding the clearing of the delirium and preventing its return. The patient will do best in a quiet setting, away from bustle and confusion, but not isolated or abandoned because isolation may worsen the delirium. Frequent attention by a relative or friend while the confusion is severe, and particularly at night, is helpful and reassuring. Visitors must be supportive and convey optimism.

Retaining or restoring familiar furnishings and memorabilia is particularly helpful if the patient is in new surroundings. Adequate lighting and the sensory stimulation provided by a television or radio are usually beneficial. Reorientation to time and date will speed recovery. Often radio or television news programs that reinforce the time and date are helpful. An old-fashioned calendar with 365 pages, each page with the day and date in large print, can be very helpful.

Medications

If the patient is agitated, the physician may prescribe a mild sedative. The use of physical restraints often worsens the agitation. Restraints are best kept for moments of absolute necessity to protect the patient from self-injury.

Notify Our Office If

- Abrupt changes in mental status occur.
- There is any suspicion of infection or injury. Patients with impaired mentation are susceptible to infection and trauma *without* manifesting the usual or expected complaints.

Disruptive Behavior

Patient and Caregiver's Guide

General Information

It is unfortunate but true that many elderly who are forced to become dependent on caregivers for some or all of their daily care respond with the development of patterns of disruptive behavior. This behavior may produce harm to the patient, caregiver, or others who live or work in close proximity to the patient. The disruptive behavior may cause physical harm or be emotionally trying or both. Disruptive behavior is often a root cause of a patient's being institutionalized. As many as one fourth of nursing home patients demonstrate this sort of behavior.

Disruptive behavior may be physical. Patients may try to physically abuse others. They may direct their abuse to their physical surroundings, damaging objects, furniture, or their room. Disruptive behavior may also take the form of resistance. The patient may refuse food, medication, or other elements of health care, such as intravenous lines or catheters. Verbal disruption by screaming or using abusive language is another pattern of disruptive behavior.

Important Points in Treatment

Management of disruptive behavior is important. The goal is to avoid the need to use physical or chemical restraints. Such management requires patience and perseverance to be successful. If there are known medical problems, these need to be treated. If the disruptive behavior involves resistance, careful attention must be paid to accommodate needs. Incontinence programs, if optimized, may forestall disruptive behavior in relationship to urination or defecation. When refusal involves food, accommodating the patient's wishes may turn refusal into acceptance. Meet with the physician and review the patient's medications. Some medication may be a part of the inducement of the disruptive behavior. If patients resist medications, alternative forms or another approach to management of the underlying problem may offer a solution.

Confinement by illness is often the initiator of disruptive events, and sudden changes in customary or scheduled events can also be a trigger.

Notify Our Office If

● The patient begins to demonstrate recurrent or consistent disruptive behavior.

Alzheimer's Disease Diagnostic Criteria

University of Washington Research Diagnostic Criteria for Primary Neuronal Degeneration of the Alzheimer's Type			

Clinical Features for Inclusion

A deterioration of general cognitive functions from a previously higher performance level compromising the ability to adapt to the environment, including:

A. Onset	Yes	No
1. Gradual progression	——	——
2. Duration of at least 6 months	——	——

B. Impairment of at least *two* of the following abilities (on the basis of performance on the Mini-Mental Status, the Wechsler Adult Intelligence Scale):

	Absent	Mild	Moderate	Severe
1. Learning	——	——	——	——
2. Attention	——	——	——	——
3. Memory	——	——	——	——
4. Orientation	——	——	——	——

C. Impairment on at least one of the following cognitive skills (on the basis of performance on the WAIS and Mini-Mental Status):

	Absent	Mild	Moderate	Severe
1. Calculation	——	——	——	——
2. Abstraction and judgment	——	——	——	——
3. Comprehension	——	——	——	——

D. Problems in at least one of the following areas (on the basis of the psychosocial examination:

	Absent	Mild	Moderate	Severe
1. Ability to work	——	——	——	——
2. Ability to relate to family	——	——	——	——
3. Ability to relate to peers	——	——	——	——
4. Ability to function socially	——	——	——	——

E. Indication of cerebral dysfunction on at least one of the following:

	Yes	No
1. Cerebral atrophy on CT scan	——	——
2. Abnormal EEG (see also exclusion criteria)	——	——

F. Ischemic score ≤ 4 (modified from Hachinski, 1978)

Feature	Possible Score	Real Score
1. Abrupt onset	2	——
2. Stepwise deterioration	1	——
3. Fluctuating course	2	——
4. Nocturnal confusion	1	——
5. Emotional lability	1	——
6. History of hypertension	1	——
7. History of strokes	2	——
8. Evidence of associated atherosclerosis	1	——
9. Focal neurologic symptoms	2	——
10. Focal neurologic signs	2	——

(*Continued on the following page*)

University of Washington Research Diagnostic Criteria for Primary Neuronal Degeneration of the Alzheimer's Type (Continued)		
Medical Exclusion Criteria	Yes	No
A. Focal neurologic signs (including EEG foci)	___	___
B. Medical history of:		
1. Myocardial infarction or chronic cardiovascular disease	___	___
2. Cardiovascular accident	___	___
3. Alcoholism or substance abuse	___	___
4. Chronic psychiatric illness	___	___
5. Syphilis	___	___
6. Brain damage sustained earlier from a known cause, eg, hypoxia	___	___
7. Chronic renal, hepatic, pulmonary, or endocrine disease	___	___
8. Parkinson's disease, Huntington's chorea, Pick's disease, or related neurologic disorders selectively affecting specific brain regions	___	___
9. Multi-infarct dementia	___	___
10. Hypertensive cardiovascular disease	___	___
C. Pseudodementias		
1. Primary manic disorder	___	___
2. Primary depressive disorder	___	___
3. Physical disorders, metabolic intoxicity, drug interaction	___	___

From Eisdorfer C, Cohen D: Research diagnostic criteria for primary neuronal degeneration of the Alzheimer type. J Fam Pract 11:553, 1980.

Mental Status Questionnaire

Mental Status Questionnaire		
Question	Response	Incorrect Responses(✓)
1. What is the name of this place?	_____	_____
2. Where is it located (address)?	_____	_____
3. What is today's date (day of month)?	_____	_____
4. What month is it?	_____	_____
5. What is the year?	_____	_____
6. How old are you?	_____	_____
7. When is your birthday?	_____	_____
8. When were you born (year)?	_____	_____
9. Who is president of the U.S.?	_____	_____
10. Who was president before him?	_____	_____
	TOTAL INCORRECT:	_____

From Kahn RL, Goldfarb AI, Pollack KM, et al: Brief objective measures for the determination of mental status in the aged. Am J Psychiatry 117:326, 1960.

Mini-Mental Status Examination

Patient _____
Examiner _____
Date _____

"MINI-MENTAL STATE"

Score   **Orientation**

(   ) What is the (year) (season) (date) (day) (month)?
(   ) Where are we: (state) (county) (town) (hospital) (floor).

Registration

(   ) Name 3 objects: 1 second to say each. Then ask the patient all 3 after you have
           said them. Give 1 point for each correct answer. Then repeat
           them until he learns all 3. Count trials and record.

                                         Trials _____

Attention and Calculation

(   ) Serial 7's. 1 point for each correct. Stop after 5 answers. Alternatively spell
      "world" backwards.

Recall

(   ) Ask for the 3 objects repeated above. Give 1 point for each correct.

Language

(   ) Name a pencil, and watch (2 points)
      Repeat the following "No ifs, ands or buts." (1 point)
      Follow a 3-stage command:
                "Take a paper in your right hand, fold it in half, and put it on the
                floor" (3 points)
      Read and obey the following:

                Close your eyes (1 point)

      Write a sentence (1 point)
      Copy design (1 point)
      Total score
      ASSESS level of consciousness
        along a continuum _____

| Alert | Drowsy | Stupor | Coma |

INSTRUCTIONS FOR ADMINISTRATION OF
MINI-MENTAL STATE EXAMINATION

Orientation

(1) Ask for the date. Then ask specifically for parts omitted, e.g., "Can you also tell me
what season it is?" One point for each correct.
(2) Ask in turn "Can you tell me the name of this hospital?" (town, county, etc.). One
point for each correct.

From Folstein MF, Folstein SE, McHugh PR: "Mini-mental state," a practical method for grading the cognitive state of patients for the clinician. J Psychiatr Res 12:189, 1975. Copyright Pergamon Press, Ltd. Reproduced with permission.

Memory Aids

General Information

Seniors do not have an exclusive option on forgetfulness, but one common feature of the aging process is the failing of short-term memory. This impairment may range in severity from simple forgetfulness to severe amnesia. In all but the most severely impaired, the use of memory aids can help to compensate for much of the memory impairment.

MEDICATIONS AND TREATMENTS

Remembering to take medication in the proper dose and at the proper time is important for the prevention and management of illness. Missed doses are a common problem in patients who do not have any unusual memory impairment, and they become a greater problem when memory begins to fail. Repeating a dose because of failure to remember that it has already been taken is also a problem. These difficulties increase with multiple drugs and the treatment of several diseases, a common occurrence in elderly patients.

The use of a simple dosing system can help the patient follow a medication schedule. For the patient:

1. Start by gathering all the medications, both prescription and nonprescription, that you take regularly. Also gather the medications that you take only as needed.
2. On a clean sheet of paper, list all of the medications or treatments across the top, using a separate column for each medication or treatment.
3. In the left margin, list each time a medication or treatment is taken, from the time of the first morning dose or treatment through the time of the last dose or treatment of the day.
4. Complete the chart by marking in each column the dose or number of pills taken for each medication at each time. When complete, you will have a daily medication schedule.
5. The next step is to try to simplify the medication schedule by grouping as many of the medications and treatments into the

same time slot as possible. Be sure to seek the help of your physician when doing this. Some medications are ineffective or even dangerous when taken together. Take a copy of this schedule on all visits to your physician. It will help the physician understand your current medication program and to ensure that any new medications or treatments are added at the best times.

For many patients, posting the simplified medication schedule in the kitchen or bathroom serves as a sufficient reminder. However, some patients need additional help to keep track of what has actually been taken each day. They should do the following:

1. Obtain one empty pill vial from your pharmacist for each time slot for which there is a medication to take or a treatment to perform.
2. Label the vial with the medicine(s) to be taken and the time it is to be taken.
3. Each morning, fill the vials with the appropriate pills. During the day, you can tell at a glance whether the dose has been taken or missed.
4. Use an alarm clock or timer as a reminder to take the next dose. Select a clock with an alarm that is simple to set and change. As one vial is emptied, reset the alarm for the time on the next vial.
5. When a treatment rather than a medication is involved, place a small square of cardboard with the name of the treatment in the vial as a reminder.

A caregiver can make a daily visit to fill the vials to ensure optimum compliance even when the patient may be alone for much of the day. This helps promote independent living without any sacrifice in treatment. When the patient is to be away from home, the proper vials should be carried in a pocket or purse to ensure that medications are taken at the proper times. Many varieties of vials and boxes designed to remind the patient to take medication at the proper time and dose can be purchased. Some hold a week's rather than a day's supply. Others have timers and alarms as reminders. Avoid selecting a gadget that is too complex to use easily and successfully. Multiple tiny hinged doors, receptacles too small to admit a finger, and complex alarms are self-defeating.

ACTIVITIES OF DAILY LIVING

Grooming and food preparation are examples of activities of daily living that involve multiple tasks, any one of which can be easily forgotten. Who among us has not at some time forgotten to shave when grooming or to put in the vanilla when baking a cake? Any momentary distraction while at morning toilette or at the kitchen counter is all that is needed. Slight memory impairment worsens this problem. Regular use of memory aids can protect against these mishaps.

Each step in daily grooming usually involves a special item: toothbrush, razor, comb, brush, lipstick, and so on. Storing these items together as a group in a drawer or on a tray, separate from other clutter, converts them into a memory aid. Begin your grooming by setting out each of the required grooming aids on a countertop or any other convenient surface in the bathroom. As each item is used, replace it in the storage drawer or on the storage tray. Everything will be used. Nothing will be forgotten. It may be necessary for the grooming aids to be set out by a caregiver for later use by the patient. This "jump-starts" the grooming process yet preserves the patient's independence and involvement in personal care.

The key to success is the use of an uncluttered environment for both storage and laying out the daily grooming aids. Clutter inevitably leads to confusion, which, in turn, defeats the purpose of the memory aid. A similar strategy is applicable to other activities of daily living, such as washing dishes, paying bills, and following recipes. Most serial or sorting tasks can be handled in this manner. The keys are:

● To use an uncluttered work area.
● To set out all items to be used.
● To return items to storage once they are used.
● To recognize that items regularly used together should be stored together.

APPOINTMENTS AND SCHEDULES

Each year there is a new "wrinkle" in ways to record appointments and schedules. Most of these products are for an office or business setting; outside a business environment, many of them lose their cleverness. None of them work unless they are used, and this means that most products are user-friendly. The two keys for a successful memory aid for appointments and schedules are:

- It must be simple to update.
- It must be accessible.

Most patients rely on a note on a slip of paper or an appointment card from their physician or dentist as their appointment reminder. These are variously hung on bulletin boards or on the front of the refrigerator. Loose papers get lost: some on the floor, others in the clutter of past appointment reminders not yet discarded. Replace these with a planner.

A full-year planner can be found in most office supply stores. This is a form of calendar that places all 12 months on a single large page with a place to write in messages for each day in the year. It is usually 2×3 feet and is available in paper or plastic. An erasable felt-tip marker is used with the plastic type. Planners cost from $5 to $10. Ten dollars is not an inconsiderable sum, but it is far less than the cost of one missed appointment.

The key to the successful use of a planner is its location. It must be where the patient sees it first thing every morning. It is best if it is reachable from the telephone. The kitchen is the usual choice, but lifestyles vary, and another room may be more appropriate for some. The patient can quickly tell whether the location is proper by noting whether he or she enters appointments on the calendar as they are made. If the patient does not, the location is wrong. Each day is marked out as it is completed with a marker. The patient will never be at a loss concerning what must be done next.

Space restrictions may require the use of a monthly or even a weekly calendar. If this is kept in order in a ring binder with the current calendar on the top, it can be left in a place that is accessible.

Driving

Patient and Caregiver's Guide

 ## General Information

Few things are as dear to each of us as our independence. The process of growing older tests our independence in many different ways. Often it seems that a driver's license is an official symbol of one's independence. In all except the largest cities, public transportation is limited. The structure of suburban America seems to require a car to complete the simple acts of daily living. No one surrenders his or her driver's license lightly.

Careful studies of accidents show that they increase for older drivers. This is true whether you consider accidents per 100,000 population or accidents per miles driven. The changes that occur with aging and its many associated diseases produce genuine impairment in some older drivers.

Several states have laws that require physicians to report impaired drivers of any age. California is the only state that currently requires specific reporting when a patient is diagnosed with dementia. Even where there are no such laws, the common law holds a physician responsible for injuries to a third person for not reporting an impaired driver. Long before impairment gets to that level, a prudent driver might assess the risk and decide to forego driving.

For drivers approaching the gray area of impairment, it should be remembered that the courts can hold a knowingly impaired driver responsible for both civil damages and criminal liability in the event of accidental injury. Prudent drivers who suspect even minimal impairment should consider the following defensive driving measures:

- Avoid driving at night. Nighttime vision may be impaired by glare and light sensitivity. If glare from oncoming lights is blinding, it is wise to forego driving at night. Careful scheduling can allow a full and active lifestyle without nighttime driving.
- Avoid busy traffic. With careful planning, chores that require driving can be done between the morning, noon, and evening

rush hours. With forethought, appointments can be accommodated during less challenging driving times.

- Group your chores. Accidents increase in frequency with miles driven. Making one trip to visit three places offers less risk than making three separate trips.
- Explore the availability of public and private transportation. Many towns offer services for senior transport. Sometimes this may be limited to transportation to a physician's appointment, but often there are resources to help with shopping trips and other activities of daily living.
- Explore the option of using taxis. Taxis may offer a reasonable, affordable option, if their use is optimized. Often by habit we bank at one location, have clothes dry-cleaned at another, shop for groceries at a third, and make a fourth trip to a drug store. Four taxi rides are expensive. Consider using a bank, dry cleaner, grocery, and pharmacy that are located together.

Mobility and involvement remain essential to good health as aging proceeds. Driving may not be the best or safest way to retain mobility.

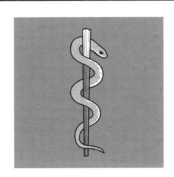
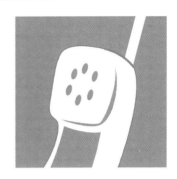

Cerebrovascular Diseases

Stroke

Patient and Caregiver's Guide

General Information

Strokes occur when there is an interruption of blood flow to part of the brain. The most common cause of the interruption of blood flow is the plugging of an artery inside or leading to the brain. The plug is most often a blood clot, or an embolus. An *embolus* is a piece of clot or other material that has broken off from somewhere else in the circulatory system. This kind of stroke, caused by interruption of blood flow, is an *ischemic stroke* and is the major cause of stroke in elderly patients. Interruption of blood flow can also occur, if bleeding (hemorrhage) occurs in or around the brain, causing a *hemorrhagic stroke*. However, this is less common in elderly patients as a cause of stroke.

Strokes may vary widely in severity. These variations occur because of differences in the duration of the interruption in blood flow, amount of brain tissue involved, and location of the affected tissue in the brain. Strokes may have only temporary effects (often called *transient ischemic attacks* [TIAs]) or may become so severe as to be life threatening. There are many gradations of severity in between.

A major stroke that causes weakness, paralysis, and difficulties with speech and thinking is readily apparent. Lesser strokes may occur and be noted only after several have occurred and there is a cumulative effect. Physical examination by your physician is often enough to begin to suspect the diagnosis. Your physician may need additional tests. These may include lumbar puncture (spinal tap), computed tomography (CT) scanning, or magnetic resonance imaging (MRI) of the head and brain (very specialized kinds of x-rays), or angiography (angiograms: x-rays of the blood vessels in the head and brain). It is also possible that problems with the heart's rhythm or with blood vessels in the neck or chest are contributory to the changes in blood flow to the brain.

Important Points in Treatment

- *Stroke is a medical emergency.*

Whenever a stroke occurs, your physician will undertake to identify quickly the cause of the stroke. This will allow the possible selection of treatment either to try to dissolve the clot or obstruction to the flow of blood or to arrest further damage to the brain and perhaps enhance the degree of recovery possible. Often when a cause cannot be identified, the use of blood thinners (anticoagulants) may be beneficial. All such therapy needs to be individualized for each patient.

Completed strokes may leave patients with a neurologic disability. The size, shape, and position of the underlying brain injury affect the extent of possible recovery. Even when the recovery of brain function is incomplete, it is possible to gain further benefit and restoration of abilities with rehabilitation. Rehabilitation involves retraining or adaptation to the neurologic defects. The nature of the brain injury sets the limits of recovery, but not all patients achieve full recovery and adaptation to deficits.

Specialized rehabilitation must be *available, accessible,* and *affordable* for the stroke patient to reach the limits of recovery. There may be a need to adjust housing and habits of living. These are challenges if one is well, and they are even greater challenges to the recovering stroke patient. Similar changes, both short-term and long-term, may be required of the caregiver. The events of stroke happen quickly, whereas recovery is a slow and often difficult task. Community programs and support groups can help both patient and caregiver in this process of accommodation.

- Successful management of recovery and rehabilitation begins at the diagnosis of stroke. It requires the enthusiastic participation of family and friends to get the maximum benefit possible.
- Therapy to prevent further strokes may involve drugs that must be taken with care and on schedule.

Notify Our Office If

- You have any sign of weakness, slurring of speech, or change in alertness. *Stroke is a medical emergency,* at least until the cause has been established and controlled.

Ischemic Stroke

Patient and Caregiver's Guide

General Information

Strokes occur when there is an interruption of blood flow to part of the brain. The most common cause of the interruption of blood flow is the plugging of an artery inside or leading to the brain. The plug is most often a blood clot, or an embolus. An *embolus* is a piece of clot or other material that has broken off from somewhere else in the circulatory system. This kind of stroke, caused by interruption of blood flow, is an *ischemic stroke* and is the major cause of stroke in elderly patients.

The importance of the diagnosis in ischemic strokes is directly related to the opportunity to limit the damage caused by the stroke and, in some cases, to reverse the effects. Strokes may vary widely in severity. These variations occur because of differences in the duration of the interruption in blood flow, amount of brain tissue involved, and location of the affected tissue in the brain. Strokes may have only temporary effects (often called *transient ischemic attacks* [TIAs]) or may become so severe as to be life threatening. There are many gradations of severity in between.

There is some urgency in proceeding with the tests to make this diagnosis. Treatment to dissolve the clot that is obstructing the blood vessel in the brain must be undertaken within 3 hours of the onset of the stroke to be optimally effective. Important diagnostic studies, in addition to the history and physical examination, include some laboratory studies and an x-ray study called *computed tomography* (CT or CAT scan) of the brain. Other studies may be required as well. Completed strokes that are not candidates for treatment by dissolving the clot may still benefit from treatment to contain the extent of the damage.

Important Points in Treatment

- *Stroke is a medical emergency.*
  Whenever a stroke occurs, your physician will undertake to identify quickly the cause of the stroke. This will allow the

possible selection of treatment either to try to dissolve the clot or obstruction to the flow of blood or to arrest further damage to the brain and perhaps enhance the degree of recovery possible. Often when a cause cannot be identified, the use of blood thinners (anticoagulants) may be beneficial. All such therapy needs to be individualized for each patient.

Completed strokes may leave patients with a neurologic disability. The size, shape, and position of the underlying brain injury affect the extent of possible recovery. Even when the recovery of brain function is incomplete, it is possible to gain further benefit and restoration of abilities with rehabilitation. Rehabilitation involves retraining or adaptation to the neurologic defects. The nature of the brain injury sets the limits of recovery, but not all patients achieve full recovery and adaptation to deficits.

Specialized rehabilitation must be *available, accessible,* and *affordable* for the stroke patient to reach the limits of recovery. There may be a need to adjust housing and habits of living. These are challenges if one is well, and they are even greater challenges to the recovering stroke patient. Similar changes, both short-term and long-term, may be required of the caregiver. The events of stroke happen quickly, whereas recovery is a slow and often difficult task. Community programs and support groups can help both patient and caregiver in this process of accommodation.

- Successful management of recovery and rehabilitation begins at the diagnosis of stroke. It requires the enthusiastic participation of family and friends to get the maximum benefit possible.
- Therapy to prevent further strokes may involve drugs that must be taken with care and on schedule.

Notify Our Office If

- You show any sign of weakness, slurring of speech, or change in alertness. *Stroke is a medical emergency,* at least until the cause is known and controlled.

Transient Ischemic Attack (TIA)

Patient and Caregiver's Guide

General Information

Transient ischemic attacks (TIAs) are small, reversible strokes. When blood flow is temporarily insufficient for part of the brain, the brain tissue will not function properly. The changes that the patient experiences are real but reversible. The affected part of the brain loses function while the blood flow is insufficient, but it does not die, which would cause permanent loss of function. The variety of symptoms produced by TIAs is large and may involve sensory or motor functions, or both. Occasionally the symptoms may be so mild and transient that they are ignored by the patient and family alike.

There are many possible causes for the decrease in blood flow. It may be caused by disease of the blood vessels within the brain or by disease of the blood vessels outside of or leading to the brain. It can be caused by a change in the heart rhythm or by heart failure that caused a decrease in the output of blood.

Important Points in Treatment

- TIA is an urgent reason to contact your physician.
- The treatment selected must match the likely cause.

Several treatment choices involve the use of potent drugs, which pose some risks themselves. Blood thinners (anticoagulants) are an example. Often treatment is confined to the use of daily doses of aspirin. Aspirin has a direct effect on the clotting of blood; thus, it can help prevent strokes. Aspirin has side effects and may cause bleeding, particularly from the gastrointestinal tract. There are other drugs with similar effects on blood clotting and may be used in place of aspirin. Plavix is one such drug. In a few cases, surgery is an option, albeit an option with some risks as well as benefits. It is important to remember that a TIA is not a disease but a symptom of underlying disease.

29

- If such attacks remain uncontrolled or poorly controlled, they may progress to a completed stroke. There is also the possibility of injury to the patient or others, if an attack occurs while the patient is driving. Diagnosis should not be delayed.

Notify Our Office If

- You have any sign of weakness, slurring of speech, or change in alertness, even if it is only transient.

Subarachnoid Hemorrhage and Intracerebral Bleeding

Patient and Caregiver's Guide

General Information

Strokes result from death of an area of brain tissue. When blood flow stops, the affected area of brain tissue loses its source of oxygen and nutrition and dies. This is an *ischemic stroke*. Bleeding into the space surrounding the brain (the subarachnoid space) or bleeding directly into the brain can also interrupt the flow of oxygen and nutrients and cause the death of brain tissue. The bleeding not only interrupts the flow of blood but also causes pressure on the tissues and can increase the pressure inside the skull, enough to be life threatening. Strokes of this sort are *hemorrhagic strokes*.

Bleeding is usually associated with a history of chronic high blood pressure. Bleeding may occur because of a weakness in a blood vessel (an aneurysm). Bleeding from an aneurysm can occur in older patients with or without high blood pressure. Control of blood pressure to normal levels is important in the prevention of both hemorrhagic and ischemic strokes. Injury, such as from falls, is another possible cause of bleeding. Treatment with blood thinners (anticoagulants), aspirin, or other anti-platelet drugs may also increase the risk of bleeding into and around the brain.

Important Points in Treatment

- *Stroke is a medical emergency.*
  Whenever a stroke occurs, your physician will undertake to identify quickly the cause of the stroke. This will allow the possible selection of treatment that may arrest the further development of brain damage and perhaps enhance the degree of recovery possible.

31

If bleeding has occurred from an aneurysm, surgery may be necessary to stop the bleeding and prevent it from occurring again. The blood pressure may need careful control if elevated. Injury that has led to bleeding may have its own special needs. If treatment to limit blood coagulation (blood thinners) becomes overzealous, coagulation factors may need to be corrected.

- Successful management of recovery and rehabilitation begins when the physician diagnoses the stroke. It requires the enthusiastic participation of family and friends to get the maximum benefit possible.

Therapy to prevent further strokes, if needed, involves drugs that must be taken with care and on schedule.

Notify Our Office If

- You have any sign of focal weakness, slurring of speech, or change in alertness. *Stroke is a medical emergency,* at least until the cause is established and controlled.

Rehabilitation After Stroke

Patient and Caregiver's Guide

General Information

After a stroke, there is a period of neurologic recovery. The extent and completeness of this recovery vary with the location and amount of damage to brain tissue. The speed with which recovery occurs varies with the same factors and with the cause of the damage to the brain. Small strokes that cause few neurologic changes may allow a patient to return quickly to normal activity. The larger the area of damaged brain tissue or the more profound the symptoms produced, the slower the recovery. Recovery after the plugging of blood flow is faster than recovery after bleeding into the brain, which, as a rule, causes more profound damage.

After hemorrhage, recovery may take many months, and full recovery may not be achieved. However, recovery of function can occur even when the brain tissue itself does not recover. This is the result of rehabilitation and retraining to find alternatives for the restoration of normal function.

Important Points in Treatment

During a period of neurologic recovery, much of the rehabilitation effort is devoted to the preservation of joint movement and maintenance of muscle strength. Restoration of bowel and bladder control is also a goal. Equally important are measures to reduce the development of complications, such as thrombosis (blood clots in the legs that can travel to the lungs), a risk in immobilized patients.

Rehabilitation activities begin as early as possible. Early efforts focus on retention of joint motion, prevention of spastic deformities, and prevention of the development of pressure sores. Rehabilitation may begin before the changes caused by the stroke have completely stabilized.

Once the neurologic changes have stabilized, rehabilitation progresses. Patients with paralysis of one side of the body begin by sitting up and then by undertaking transfer (getting from bed to chair and back). Various exercises, including standing, are gradually introduced according to each patient's needs. Some patients need braces to help their walking; others may require speech therapy.

Beyond these first steps, all rehabilitation is determined by individual needs. As discharge from rehabilitation approaches, an evaluation is done to determine the need for structural changes in and around the home to facilitate the maximum level of independent living.

Rehabilitation is a slow process that works best in a positive atmosphere of support from family and friends.

- Successful management of recovery and rehabilitation begins when the physician diagnoses the stroke. It requires the enthusiastic participation of family and friends to get the maximum benefit possible.

Aspirin and Other Clot-Preventing Drugs in the Prevention of Stroke

Patient and Caregiver's Guide

General Information

Strokes occur when there is an interruption of blood flow to part of the brain. The most common cause of the interruption of blood flow is the plugging of an artery inside or leading to the brain. The plug is most often a blood clot, or an embolus. An *embolus* is a piece of clot or other material that has broken off from somewhere else in the circulatory system. This kind of stroke, caused by interruption of blood flow, is an *ischemic stroke* and is the major cause of stroke in elderly patients. Transient ischemic attacks (TIAs) are small, reversible strokes. When blood flow is temporarily insufficient for part of the brain, the brain tissue will not function properly. The changes that the patient experiences are real but reversible. The affected part of the brain loses function while the blood flow is insufficient, but it does not die, which would cause permanent loss of function.

In an effort to prevent additional strokes or, if the patient has only TIAs, to prevent the development of stroke, aspirin is administered. Aspirin impairs blood clotting by its effect on a tiny blood element called a *platelet*. Platelets are essential for normal clotting of blood. Other anti-platelet agents include Dipyridamole, ticlopidine, and clopidogrel.

Important Points in Treatment

These are potent drugs used for the modification of blood clotting. Individual patients vary in their sensitivity to aspirin. Often it takes a higher dose of aspirin to achieve the desired effect than is required for the prevention of heart attacks. The usual dose of 325 mg of aspirin daily may be modified for some patients.

Additional medicines, such as Persantine or Trental, may be added in some cases to potentiate (increase) the effect of the aspirin.

Large doses of aspirin may be associated with the development of bruising or the onset of bleeding from the gastrointestinal tract. These complications may limit the use and effectiveness of aspirin in some patients.

 ## Notify Our Office If

- There is any evidence of bleeding while on aspirin therapy. Bleeding may occur in the urine, in the stool (as bright-red blood, maroon-colored stools, or black stools), or in the skin as bruising.

Swallowing Difficulty After Stroke (Dysphagia)

Patient and Caregiver's Guide

General Information

Strokes occur when there is an interruption of blood flow to part of the brain. The most common cause of the interruption of blood flow is the plugging of an artery inside or leading to the brain. The plug is most often a blood clot, or an embolus. An *embolus* is a piece of clot or other material that has broken off from somewhere else in the circulatory system. This kind of stroke, caused by interruption of blood flow, is an *ischemic stroke* and is the major cause of stroke in elderly patients.

Strokes may impair function, and it is common for these patients to have difficulty swallowing. Patients may have difficulty with food or with food and secretions, such as saliva. The impairment of swallowing may cause choking if the food, drink, or secretions enter the windpipe. Food, drink, or secretions entering the windpipe is called *aspiration*. Aspiration may lead to the development of pneumonia because of foreign materials entering the lung.

Difficulty swallowing (dysphagia) may occur only during the acute period of the stroke, but it may also become a permanent disability. After recovery has begun, if difficulty with swallowing persists, a swallowing test may be performed to determine the extent of the swallowing disability. This is often done with the help of an x-ray examination at the time of swallowing.

Important Points in Treatment

- Swallowing difficulties after stroke require treatment to protect the patient's lungs and to provide nutrition.
- Early during the course of the stroke, the doctor may place a tube through the nose and into the stomach to provide a safe way to give fluids, nutrition, and medications.
- The swallowing study will often determine that the thickening of foods will facilitate swallowing. Special thickeners are available for this purpose.

- If swallowing poses a risk of aspiration of food or fluids into the lung, alternative approaches to feeding may be required. These may include the use of a nasojejunal feeding tube, the placement of a gastric (stomach) or jejunal (small bowel) feeding tube, or the use of total parental nutrition (feeding solely through the vein).

- A nasojejunal feeding tube is a thin plastic tube placed through the nose and positioned in the upper small intestine. It may be used to give the patient food, fluids, and medicines. These tubes are thin and soft and are unlike the larger tubes placed into the stomach after major surgery. One does become accustomed to them. They are not irritating.

- Gastric (stomach) or jejunal (small intestinal) feeding tubes are placed through the skin of the abdomen and into the stomach or intestine. They provide direct access for feedings, fluids, and drugs. They may be placed surgically by operation. This is minor surgery that may be done with the use of a local anesthetic. They may also be placed through the use of an endoscope. An endoscopically placed tube is called a percutaneous endoscopic gastrostomy (PEG) tube if it is placed in the stomach, or a percutaneous endoscopic jejunostomy (PEJ) tube if it is placed in the jejunum. These tubes are not permanent and may be removed, if the patient later recovers adequate swallowing function.

- Total parenteral nutrition or feeding entirely through the vein requires the surgical placement of a tube in a large vein. It is the most expensive option, and there is some risk of infection.

Choice of the most appropriate solution for feeding when there is difficulty swallowing is a matter to discuss with your physician.

CHAPTER 3

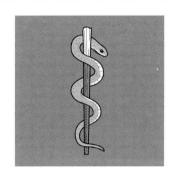
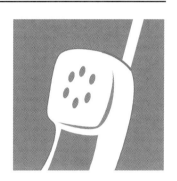

Tremors

Parkinsonian Tremor

Patient and Caregiver's Guide

General Information

Parkinson's disease, sometimes called *paralysis agitans,* is a problem caused by changes in a portion of the brain. The cause of Parkinson's disease is not well understood. A few cases occur after viral infections, but the interval between infection and onset of Parkinson's disease may be very long. Parkinson's disease affects older people, with most cases occurring after age 50. The most visible sign of the disease is a tremor or shaking. Often the tremor will affect only one side of the body at the beginning. The tremor is but one manifestation of the underlying problem. Patients with Parkinson's disease also experience muscular rigidity, slowness of movement, and disturbed posture.

Parkinsonian tremor may involve one or both hands. The tremor is present at rest and is less evident with movement. It is a rhythmic movement. In the fingers, this produces a rubbing of the fingers over the thumb, which is often called a *pill-rolling tremor.* The tremor can also affect the arms, legs, head, and mouth.

Important Points In Treatment

A variety of agents are useful in the treatment of various stages of Parkinson's disease. Education and support are essential elements of the treatment at the beginning of Parkinson's disease. Support includes the participation of the family and often will involve support groups. A program of regular exercise is important for the patient's physical well-being and helps to promote emotional stability as well.

In addition, a number of other health problems can simulate Parkinson's disease, and a number of drugs can have parkinsonian side effects. The physician will first evaluate the patient to ensure that drug effects or other diseases are not underlying the development of the tremor. Treatment is individualized to meet the specific needs of each patient. Selection of treatment will vary with the stage of the disease and the age of the patient.

- Treatment of Parkinson's disease depends on careful dosing with selected drugs. Memory aids should be used to ensure that the proper numbers of pills are taken regularly.
- Parkinson's disease may cause some unsteadiness. Adjust the household environment to reduce the likelihood of falls. This might include rearrangement of furniture, removal of throw rugs, installation of strategically placed handholds, and use of a cane or walker.
- The medications used may have side effects that change the posture or cause movements that are different from the tremor. The medications may also produce mental changes, such as confusion.
- Depression may also occur with Parkinson's disease. It may interfere with treatment and thus may need treatment itself.
- Daytime sleepiness may well be a problem. This can be a part of the Parkinson's disease or can be related to some of the drug therapy.

Surgical Treatment

The disability caused by Parkinson's disease has made it the focus of much research. A number of surgical operations have been tried. These have proven to be of help in only a minority of patients. Some forms of therapy for parkinsonism remain experimental and are controversial. Your physician is your best guide to the opportunities that might be suited to your individual needs.

Two general kinds of operations are performed for the treatment of Parkinson's disease: (1) the destruction of very selective tiny areas of the brain and (2) the implantation of other tissues into the brain. In addition, there is an operation that involves placement of an electronic device to stimulate selected areas of the brain.

The effectiveness of the operations that involve destruction of tiny selective areas of the brain depends on the ability of the surgeon to find exactly the right location within the brain. The problem is the difficulty in locating this spot. With new tools available to make images of the brain, this surgical treatment is once again being used. It is most useful for patients with a tremor on only one side of the body. For these patients, it can be effective, but complications occur in 1 out of every 10 patients.

There have been many newspaper reports of the implantation of tissues, particularly fetal tissue, into the brain to relieve the changes of Parkinson's disease. Early studies are promising, but this is still a research operation and not recommended or generally available.

A trial is being conducted to look at the use of tiny electrodes implanted in the brain to allow for the stimulation of an area that, in turn, will cause the tremor to subside. This operation is also under research study and is not recommended or generally available.

The most effective treatment for Parkinson's disease is still drug therapy. In a few patients who fail to respond to drug therapy or who cannot take the most useful drugs, the possibility of surgical treatment may be considered.

Notify Our Office If

- You have complications of drug treatment. These include blurring of vision, difficulty with urination, and confusion. Drug treatment for Parkinson's disease must be tailored to each patient. The various drugs used each have side effects that, if neglected, can result in complications. Visits to the physician may need to be more frequent during the initial period of therapy. Once treatment is established, regular but less-frequent visits will be necessary.
- You notice the sudden onset of intervals of daytime sleepiness.

Benign Essential Tremor and Senile Tremor

Patient and Caregiver's Guide

General Information

Tremor, or shaking movements, may have many causes. *Essential tremor* is not caused by an underlying disease; thus, it does not mark a progressive or debilitating problem. Most cases begin before age 25. However, variety called *senile tremor* begins in old age. This tremor involves the arms, hands, and face. It usually starts in, and it may remain confined to, one side of the body. It tends to progress slowly. Initially the tremor occurs only with movement, but as it advances, it begins to occur at rest. The tremor is not disabling and does not impair activity. This is in contrast to essential tremor, which occurs at a younger age and can progress to the point of physical disability and interfere with socialization.

Important Points In Treatment

The use of some medications, such as sedatives, may reduce the tremor, but the benefits are mild and the side effects may be disturbing. No treatment is effective in reversing the development of senile tremor. Single doses of some medications may help by providing lessening of the tremor for a short interval, which may help the patient participate socially.

Tardive Dyskinesia

Patient and Caregiver's Guide ■ ■ ■

General Information

Tardive dyskinesia is the name given to a motion disorder that is an occasional problem among the elderly. It is the result of drug therapy, in effect, a side effect of a selected list of drugs. These include the following drugs and drug families:

- Phenothiazines
- L-DOPA
- Phenytoin
- Reglan
- Cocaine
- Amphetamines
- Tricyclic antidepressants

The side effect of the drugs is a series of involuntary movements. Most commonly these will involve the mouth and other facial movements, but the extremities and even breathing can be involved. Involvement usually occurs only after prolonged treatment. Other than taking the drug(s), age is the most significant risk factor for the development of tardive dyskinesia.

Important Points In Treatment

Prevention of the development of this disorder is most important. Unlike many other drug reactions and side effects of drugs, tardive dyskinesia often will not disappear after the offending drug is no longer being taken.

It is important to take these drugs only when medically necessary. If there are any signs of unusual tremors or movements, particularly of the face and mouth, you should notify your physician immediately.

Call Our Office If

- You notice any signs of *unusual tremors* or *movements,* particularly of the face and mouth.
- You notice any *unusual tremors* or *movements* of the arms, hands, legs, or feet.

CHAPTER 4

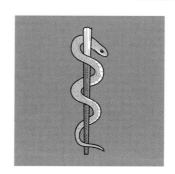
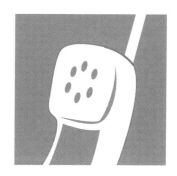

Sleep Disturbances

Insomnia

General Information

Insomnia is not exclusive to elderly patients, but it is a common accompaniment of the aging process. Insomnia is unsatisfactory sleep. Some patients have trouble falling asleep. Others have difficulty remaining asleep, either frequently waking at night or waking early in the morning. The result is daytime fatigue and often daytime naps, which compound the problem. Often the insomnia is transient and seems related to an acute stressful circumstance. Under some circumstances, this insomnia can convert to a chronic problem.

Sleep patterns frequently change with aging. Daytime naps often compensate for nocturnal awakenings. Tiredness then prompts an early bedtime, which is spoiled by a long interval waiting for sleep to come. This becomes a vicious circle.

It is often possible for a physician to determine the pattern of sleep disturbance from an interview alone, but the interview may need to include the sleeping partner, if there is one. The origins of some disturbances occur while the patient is sleeping and is thus unaware of that aspect of the problem. Whenever more careful observation is necessary, a referral to a sleep clinic may be made. Sleep clinics record the characteristics of a patient's sleep pattern on machines that help to judge the depth of sleep.

Important Points In Treatment

Management of insomnia begins with attention given to an optimum sleep environment. Your physician can help resolve some problems that lead to insomnia, but your cooperation and participation are necessary to correct emerging bad sleep habits. Your physician will look for diseases that may disturb sleep. Pain from musculoskeletal problems, even if mild, may be enough to disturb sleep. Nocturnal shortness of breath from heart and lung problems may also disturb sleep. Bowel and bladder problems are other common causes of sleep disturbance. These problems

49

need not be severe and may be little noticed during the day but can become nagging destroyers of sleep at night. You must tell your physician of these problems to get help with their control.

Some medications can cause sleeplessness, an effect that can often be avoided by adjusting the timing of the medications. Similarly, if you often wake with an urge to urinate, drink fluids earlier in the evening rather than just before bedtime to allow uninterrupted sleep. However, this should be a shift in drinking habits, not discontinuance of adequate fluid intake.

Smoking tobacco may interfere with the ability to fall asleep. Sedatives (sleeping pills) should be used only under the guidance of your physician.

Several rules are important to follow:

- Maintain as regular a sleep-wake schedule as is possible.
- Avoid daytime naps.
- Always go to bed with the intention of going to sleep. Do not read or watch television in bed. If you cannot sleep, get up and engage in some activity until you tire.
- Approach bedtime in a restful state of mind. Avoid excitement just before bedtime.
- Adjust things to feel right—the right bed, right level of darkness, right level of quiet, and right temperature.
- Do not go to bed hungry or inebriated or immediately after exercise or an emotional event.
- Do not go to bed too early. Do not hesitate to sleep late in the morning.
- Avoid smoking, heavy meals, or highly spiced meals close to your bedtime.
- Use sedatives only under the guidance of your physician.

 # Notify Our Office If

- You experience excessive daytime tiredness with frequent naps. Sleep disturbances may be subtle.

Insomnia

General Information

Insomnia is not exclusive to elderly patients, but it is a common accompaniment of the aging process.

Insomnia is unsatisfactory sleep. Some patients have trouble falling asleep. Others have difficulty remaining asleep, either frequently waking at night or waking early in the morning. The result is daytime fatigue and often daytime naps, which compound the problem. Often the insomnia is transient and seems related to an acute stressful circumstance. Under some circumstances, this insomnia can convert to a chronic problem.

Sleep patterns frequently change with aging. Daytime naps often compensate for nocturnal awakenings. Tiredness then prompts an early bedtime, which is spoiled by a long interval before sleep comes. This becomes a vicious circle.

Sleep disturbances cause different problems for caregivers than they do for patients. They are a major cause for institutionalization.

Important Points In Treatment

Management of insomnia begins with attention given to an optimum sleep environment.

- Establish a regular bedtime for the patient. Do not have the patient spend time in bed, except to sleep.
- Limit the number and duration of daytime naps.
- Adjust things to feel right—the right bed, right level of darkness, right level of quiet, and right temperature.
- Do not send the patient to bed hungry or inebriated or immediately after exercise or an emotional event.
- Avoid administering sedatives (sleeping pills) except as directed by the patient's physician.
- Avoid giving a heavy meal or a highly spiced meal immediately before bedtime.

Some medications can cause sleeplessness, an effect that can often be avoided by adjusting the timing of the medications. Seek the counsel of the patient's physician in this regard. Similarly, if the patient wakes with an urge to urinate, offer fluids earlier in the evening rather than just before bedtime to allow uninterrupted sleep. However, this should be a shift in drinking habits, not discontinuance of adequate fluid intake.

Work with the patient's physician to find a solution that avoids drugged sleep whenever possible. Sedatives should be used only under the guidance of the patient's physician. Take special care to prevent falls at night when the patient is partially sedated. Sedatives may cause confusion and thus the inability to remember what other medicines have been taken.

Notify Our Office If

- The patient's insomnia persists beyond a week. For a few people with insomnia, associated disease is the cause of the sleeplessness.
- The patient experiences excessive daytime tiredness with frequent naps. Sleep disturbances may be subtle.

Somnolence

Patient and Caregiver's Guide ▪ ▪ ▪

General Information

Somnolence is not exclusive to elderly patients, but it is a common accompaniment of the aging process.

Two medical problems occur with somnolence, or excessive sleeping. Obstructive sleep apnea is the most common. This means a stopping of breathing that lasts for more than 10 seconds by obstruction of the passages in the upper airway. This occurs in people who are overweight and who have high blood pressure. In younger patients, it is more common in men than in women, but with advancing years, more women are sufferers. Loud snoring alone is not a disease problem; however, it may be disturbing to a sleeping partner.

With obstructive sleep apnea, breathing stops, but the patient continues to struggle to breathe. Breathing restarts with a snort or a grunt rather than the gradual increase associated with periodic breathing. The patient remains unaware of these breathing problems, although he or she may note some fatigue during the day. Daytime sleepiness and confusion on awakening also occur.

Untreated sleep apnea may have serious health consequences. High blood pressure and other cardiovascular problems may be more common with this sleep disturbance. The nonmedical consequences of sleepiness that result from sleep apnea may be important as well. Impairment of the ability to operate a car may result in the loss of one's driver's license. Your physician may be legally required to report this impairment.

Important Points In Treatment

Sleep apnea is a serious problem. Stroke, heart attacks, decreased kidney function, and sudden death occur with sleep apnea. The diagnosis and management of sleep apnea are done at centers for the study of sleep disorders.

Treatment may involve changes in one's lifestyle. Weight loss is important. Restriction of the use of tobacco, alcohol, and many drugs can also be helpful. Treatment of conditions causing nasal congestion or inflammation may also be necessary.

Notify Our Office If

● You snore loudly with difficult or interrupted breathing.

Disorders of the Sleep-Wake Cycle

Patient and Caregiver's Guide

General Information

Disorders of the sleep-wake cycle are not exclusive to elderly patients, but they are common accompaniments of the aging process.

All humans live with a normal, almost 24-hour rhythm called the *circadian rhythm*. The sleep-wake cycle is part of this rhythm. Disturbances in the control of the rhythm occur with increased frequency as individuals grow older. The changes that may occur include:

- Delayed sleep onset—patients fall asleep 4 to 5 hours after the desired time and often oversleep the same number of hours. The actual duration of sleep time may be normal.
- Advanced sleep phase—patients fall asleep earlier than the desired bedtime but also awaken earlier than desired. The actual duration of sleep time may be normal. Daytime sleepiness may be a problem in these patients.
- Irregular sleep-wake phase—patients have no real schedule.

Anyone can experience a temporary shift in or an abnormality of the sleep-wake cycle, but when a changed sleep-wake cycle pattern persists for more than a week, it should prompt a visit to your physician.

Important Points In Treatment

Abnormalities of the sleep-wake cycle take different forms, but there are a few general guides for management. Management begins with attention being given to an optimum sleep environment. Your physician can help resolve some problems, but your cooperation and participation are necessary to correct emerging bad sleep habits.

Several rules are important to follow:

- Always go to bed with the intention of going to sleep. Do not read or watch television in bed. If you cannot sleep, get up and engage in some activity until you tire.
- Approach bedtime in a restful state of mind. Avoid excitement just before bedtime.
- Adjust things to feel right—the right bed, right level of darkness, right level of quiet, and right temperature.
- Do not go to bed hungry or inebriated or immediately after exercise or an emotional event.

If you wake with an urge to urinate, drink fluids earlier in the evening rather than just before bedtime to allow uninterrupted sleep. However, this should be a shift in drinking habits, not discontinuance of adequate fluid intake.

Sedatives (sleeping pills) should be used only under the guidance of your physician. Take special care to prevent falls at night when partially sedated. Sedatives may cause confusion and thus an inability to remember what other medicines have been taken.

Notify Our Office If

- You experience excessive daytime tiredness with frequent naps. Sleep disturbances may be subtle.

Sleepwalking

General Information

Sleepwalking is a real occurrence not just a clever idea for a novel. The proper medical name for this type of parasomnia is *arousal disorder*. Individuals who are sleepwalkers can engage in very complicated behavior yet remain completely unaware of what they have done. It is possible for them to injure themselves or others during a sleepwalking interval. Evidence that an individual is a sleepwalker should be taken seriously. Such behavior often requires referral to a specialist.

Important Points In Treatment

Sleepwalking is not usually associated with problems of insomnia or with excessive sleepiness. Treatment is largely directed toward preventing the sleepwalker from engaging in activities that can lead to injury either to themselves or to others.

Notify Our Office If

- There is any suggestion that sleepwalking has occurred.

Jet Lag

General Information

Jet lag occurs when a person makes a long flight over many time zones. Such a flight disturbs what is called the *body's internal clock*. The result may be no more than sleepiness coming on at an inconvenient time; however, many people experience other difficulties in association with jet lag, including memory difficulties, dizziness, generalized weakness, difficulty with concentration, and even momentary disorientation and confusion on awakening. Generally these symptoms manifest in the older traveler.

The Problem

When one flies east the most notable problem is falling asleep at bedtime in the new time zone. With westward travel, the difficulty is early awakening. North–south flights do not cross time zones and generally cause no problems.

The underlying difficulty is a dissociation between your body's internal clock and the local time in the new time zone. Your body tells you that it is or isn't time to go to sleep or wake up, and this does not match the clock time in your new time zone. Gradually your body clock will adjust to the new clock time, but this adjustment is a relatively slow process and may not move more than an hour per day. This adjustment may be speeded up by controlling exposure to light, by using the drug melatonin, or by diet and physical activity.

Important Points In Treatment

Slowing travel markedly reduces the jet lag effect. If it is possible to break up the trip into intervals, this should be done. Some pre-planning will also help. If you are flying east, then, for several days before the trip starts, try going to bed earlier in the evening and rising earlier in the morning. When you rise in the morning make sure that you are exposed to bright lights. This will speed the adjustment of the internal clock by several days. If flying west, try to stay up later and sleep in the morning. If you do rise in the morning briefly to go to the bathroom, try to avoid bright lights and then return to bed. This sort of preparation can make limited time shifts of 2 or 3 hours negligible.

If your trip is over many time zones but is to be of very short duration, 3 days or less, consider not shifting your own personal clock. Manage your appointments as though you were in your own time zone and follow your home sleep pattern as much as possible.

If your trip is for a long stay, then try to arrive several days before an important appointment or meeting. Permit time for your internal clock to adjust itself. This will help you to enjoy and participate in the purpose of your travel, whether business or vacation.

Short naps during the adjustment period are not harmful to the process of adjustment of your body's internal clock. Long naps of 4 or more hours will interfere with this process of adjustment. A short nap can restore your alertness for a meeting or an event. Drugs to promote sleep or alertness often have negative effects and should be avoided.

The drug melatonin is widely marketed to help speed the adjustment of the body's internal clock. Its use is controversial, and the drug does not have the approval of the Food and Drug Administration (FDA) for this purpose. There are also elaborate programs and devices to control or promote exposure to light to attempt to speed the body clock's adjustment. These may be fun to try and are harmless.

Call Our Office If

- You are planning a long trip over multiple time zones and wish to avoid or diminish the problem of jet lag.
- You are planning a long trip over many time zones and are concerned about the timing of your medications.

CHAPTER 5

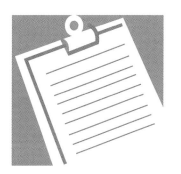 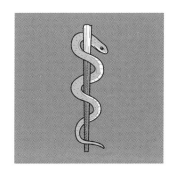 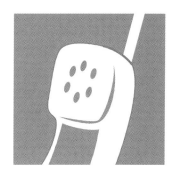

Falls and Instability

Falls and Instability

Patient and Caregiver's Guide

General Information

Falls are a major cause of both disability and death in senior citizens. They occur frequently. More than one third of people over age 65 have at least one fall each year. After a fall, elderly patients frequently voluntarily restrict their activity because they fear another fall. The occurrence of falls is a strong predictor of nursing home placement. Reduction in exercise leads to further weakness that, in turn, increases the risk of another fall, a vicious circle. Older patients need protection while walking after a fall to allow them to retain an adequate level of physical fitness.

Injuries sustained in a fall may range from trivial bruises to life-threatening trauma. Head injuries and fractures of long bones lead the list of serious outcomes. There may be a delay in the onset of the effects of head injury.

Several medical problems may predispose a patient to suffer a fall. Visual changes that decrease visual acuity, particularly at night or in the dark, increase the chances of a fall. Neurologic problems that cause weakness or affect stability and balance also set the stage for a fall. More serious medical problems, such as stroke, seizures, bleeding with associated anemia, and heart disease, particularly abnormalities in heart rate and rhythm, can lead to falls. Any medical problem that causes debility is a factor. With these serious diseases the prime focus of concern is the major health problem, but a fall can immeasurably compound these problems. A fall adds to the acute problem and prolongs recovery.

Important Points In Treatment

All falls merit some degree of evaluation. If there has been a health risk, your physician should be involved in the evaluation and any needed treatment. If health and limb remain intact, there is still a concern about why the fall occurred and how to prevent more falls. Your physician can help evaluate health-related causes, but you must evaluate environmental causes in the home.

The environment is responsible for more than one third of all falls. Improper lighting, inadequate handholds, unstable furniture, loose rugs, and uneven floors all pose risks. Just as it is possible to childproof a house for a toddler, it is possible to "fallproof" a house for yourself. The shortest route from one place in the house to another may not be the safest. Always take the safest route. Remove hazards even if they are heirlooms. Rugs, throw rugs, and furniture are all avoidable hazards. Stairs should be supplemented with handholds for safety. Make sure that light switches are available at the doors or, if possible, outside the doors to dark rooms. Use night-lights freely. Adjust lighting so that it is even and bright enough to reveal obstacles.

Furnishings should be sturdy and stable to permit them to provide necessary support, if they are leaned upon. The bathroom has the potential of being particularly hazardous. Nonskid mats are important both inside and outside the bath. Towel racks do not substitute for handrails. Leave the bathroom door unlocked or at least able to be opened from the outside.

Time and other efforts spent maintaining safe mobility are more than compensated by savings in pain and disability and by an improved quality of life.

Recent studies have shown that a fall occurring on a cement floor is more likely to cause injury than a fall that occurs on a hardwood floor covered with a rug. These become guidelines if the patient decides that the time has come to move to a new environment.

The interval after a fall is a critical one for the patient. It is the period of time when the support of the caregiver is essential to help the patient retain a willingness to remain active. Fear of another fall can be an inhibitor of a patient's remaining fully active.

Notify Our Office If

- You have a fall. All falls merit some degree of evaluation. If there has been a health risk, your physician should be involved in the evaluation and treatment indicated.
- You have any sign of confusion after a fall. There may be a delay in the onset of the consequences of head injury.

Shoes and Falls

Patient and Caregiver's Guide

General Information

With advancing age the risk of a fall increases. A fall may not only produce an injury but may also result in the limitation of activities that will impair the quality of life and the ability to engage fully in the ordinary activities of living. Selection of footwear is an important factor in the prevention of falls.

It is a common observation that well-fitting athletic shoes or sturdy, well-fitting leather shoes provide safer, surer footing than scuffs, slippers, or slip-ons. Careful study has shown this not to be true. Most falls occur to people who are soundly shod. It is true that well-fitting shoes firmly laced are important preventives. Loose, floppy, or ill-fitting footwear adds to the risk of instability, which may lead to a fall.

Important Points in Prevention

Equally important or perhaps more important is the selection of shoes with soles that are safely usable in your own environment. Soles must be matched to the floor surface on which they tread. Shoes with smooth soles—leather, rubber, or plastic—may be equally slick and unsteady on carpet or bare floor. Shoes may come with smooth soles or the soles may be worn smooth. Shoes with lug soles, particularly rubber lug soles, do well on smooth floors but may catch in fibers of the carpet nap, particularly if the carpet has a thick pile. Many well-constructed, expensive athletic shoes feature such a lugged construction. Shoes with a textured rubber or composition sole are a better compromise for steady footing.

Many athletic shoes, particularly those designed for running and active sports, have a rubber toe cap. These toe caps are designed to provide traction as the athlete pushes forward at a run. They also tend to catch in carpet pile and may prompt a spill. This is a particular problem with patients who have difficulty picking up their feet as they walk and, as a result, they shuffle.

Shoes designed for walking as exercise often offer the best balance of a sole designed for nonslip traction without lugs or caps that trip you up.

Lace-up shoes will permit a careful adjustment for a snug but not restrictive fit. This is of importance with feet prone to swelling or with deforming arthritis. Laces can be hard to handle. Velcro closure or elastic laces are available and offer the compromise of permitting adjustment when needed without the need for retying every time you put on your shoes. Elastic-laced shoes may be slipped into with the aid of a long-handled shoe horn.

Notify Our Office If

- You have a fall. All falls merit some degree of evaluation. If there has been a health risk, your physician should be involved in the evaluation and treatment indicated.
- You have any sign of confusion after a fall. There may be a delay in the onset of the consequences of head injury.

CHAPTER 6

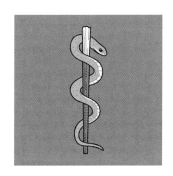
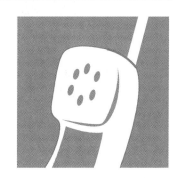

Special Senses: Vision, Hearing, Taste, and Smell

Presbyopia

Patient and Caregiver's Guide

General Information

Everyone experiences a change in the eyes with aging. The result of this change is the loss of the ability of the lens of the eye to adapt for near vision. This loss of accommodation is called *presbyopia*.

Presbyopic change begins in people in their early 40s and usually stabilizes around age 65. You can correct near vision by using magnifying lenses, that is, common reading glasses. Presbyopic change is gradual and slowly progressive over a period as long as several decades, and a change in your reading lenses to a greater strength is needed every few years until the presbyopia stabilizes.

Important Points In Treatment

Presbyopia occurs with the aging of the lens of the eye. Very little can be done short of using corrective lenses to remedy this problem.

The appropriate management of presbyopia is the use of magnifying lenses for reading. If you already wear eyeglasses, then bifocals or, as the presbyopia progresses, trifocals can restore near and middle vision. The presbyopic change progresses for a decade or so and then stabilizes.

Notify Our Office If

- You have a recurrent headache while reading. The visual changes that occur with presbyopia are gradual in onset. Headaches secondary to eyestrain may precede more obvious changes, such as blurred vision for near objects.

Cataracts

General Information

Cataracts are areas of clouding or opacity on the lens of the eye. If they are large enough or are located strategically in the visual path, they may reduce visual acuity. Although some cataracts that form are not part of the aging process and may occur at any age, there are cataracts that come with growing old. The first of the age-related changes may begin as early as age 40. The speed with which cataracts develop and their extent remain highly variable from person to person. The development of cataracts often causes a problem with glare.

Important Points In Treatment

The treatment of cataracts is by surgical removal of the clouded lens and its replacement, usually with a lens implant. As with all surgery, there are risks and complications. When the visual clouding caused by the cataract outweighs the risks, surgery may be necessary. Risk factors include other eye diseases; also, other health problems may preclude surgery. Your physician will help you sort through these risks in a meaningful fashion. Cataract surgery may be an outpatient or short-stay procedure.

Notify Our Office If

● Glare is unusually bothersome, especially at night. The development of cataracts often causes a problem with glare.

Glare

General Information

Any bright light shining into the eye causes glare and reduces visual acuity. Changes that occur in the eye as it ages allow glare to occur more easily. As one grows older, it is not uncommon for small opacities to develop in the eye, particularly on the lens. These are small cataracts. These are often too small to cause any visual impairment, but when light shines directly into the eye, the opacities can cause the light to scatter, much as motes of dust in the air scatter a beam of sunlight. It is scattered light that causes glare.

Glare is usually a problem at night, especially when one is driving. In the dark, the pupil of the eye dilates, exposing more of the lens in the eye for the passage of light. This increases the chances of light hitting the opacities and then scattering. Oncoming headlights can cause blinding flashes of light that can affect the ability to see.

Important Points In Treatment

If you have good visual acuity except when facing bright lights, there is little that can be done. Not looking directly into oncoming lights will help, but if the glare is severe, avoiding night driving may be the only prudent solution.

A few patients suffer daytime problems with glare. This is usually a result of a larger opacity located more centrally in the light path through the eye. Again, these opacities may not be severe enough to impair vision unless a bright light is shining into the eye.

Daytime glare is a more difficult problem to manage. Wearing sunglasses often helps. Management with drugs to contract the pupil should be under the direction of an ophthalmologist.

The caregiver should ensure that light is even and from multiple sources so that the patient gets adequate light levels without glare. Curtains or blinds should be adjusted to diffuse sunlight and to prevent direct illumination. Shiny surfaces, waxed floors, and reflective fixtures all look attractive but add to the problem of glare.

Notify Our Office If

- You have a particular problem with glare at night, or if glare is a complaint while driving at night.

Low Vision

Patient and Caregiver's Guide

General Information

Between the extremes of vision that are normal (or that can be corrected to near normal with eyeglasses) and blindness, there is a problem called *low vision*. Every effort should be made to ensure that all reversible aspects of visual change are treated in patients who suffer from low vision. The vision that remains forms the baseline from which the patient and the caregiver must work.

Important Points In Treatment

The principal resources for the treatment and management of low vision are a low-vision specialist and a low-vision clinic. Many devices and resources are available to help vision-impaired patients. Most people are familiar with large-type books, recordings, and descriptive television. Many other devices are also available to help compensate for vision loss, and there is a need not only to find them but to train vision-impaired patients in their proper use. It is in this area that low-vision specialists and low-vision clinics offer particular assistance.

Much can be done to modify the home surroundings to allow the patient with low vision to adapt. Adequate light evenly distributed to avoid glare is important. One can substitute color and contrast for bland backgrounds to help with the identification of each room. It helps for a patient to know that blue is the bedroom, pink is the living room, white is the bathroom, green is the kitchen, and so on. Contrast may also help the patient around within the room (e.g., the color of the furniture and furniture coverings should contrast with the color of the floors, carpets, and walls). Similarly, china, glassware, and cutlery should contrast with the tabletop, tablecloth, or placemat and with one another. Transparent glass tabletops simply disappear for a patient with low vision. Selection of colors for their contrast rather than their aesthetics may produce unusual combinations, but it also keeps the objects visible to an individual with low vision.

Night-lights, glowing switches, and other lighted or glow-in-the-dark guides can aid a patient in getting from the bed to the bathroom or from the bed to the kitchen at night. Where possible, it may be desirable to mount light switches outside the room so that the patient does not need to enter a darkened room and grope for a switch. Switches are available that permit such a change without the need for rewiring. With thought and imagination, independence in living can be restored to patients with low vision.

Summary

- Much can be done to modify the home surroundings to allow the patient with low vision to adapt.
- Selection of colors for their contrast keeps objects visible to an individual with low vision.
- With thought and imagination, independence in living can be restored to patients with low vision.

Glaucoma

Patient and Caregiver's Guide

General Information

The condition in which the fluids within the eye develop a higher-than-normal pressure is called *glaucoma*. If glaucoma is not treated, the increased pressure is transmitted to the optic nerves and can produce an irreversible loss of vision or even complete blindness. Glaucoma causes 10% of the blindness that occurs in the United States. Although glaucoma is not a result of an aging change in the eye, it does occur with increasing frequency after age 40; it occurs in 4% of the population by age 65 and in 15% by age 80. African Americans are far more commonly affected than whites.

Of the several different varieties of glaucoma, open-angle glaucoma causes most of the problems in elderly patients. Open-angle glaucoma usually produces no symptoms for a long period. Unlike other varieties of glaucoma, it does not cause pain in the eye. Gradually, there is a loss of part of what physicians call the *visual field*. This usually happens in both eyes, and it may develop so slowly that you remain unaware of the visual field loss until it becomes advanced and irreversible.

Some patients are at particular risk for glaucoma. These include patients with a family history of glaucoma (a parent, brother, or sister) and patients who are receiving long-term therapy with steroid medications. Patients with high blood pressure, diabetes, and near-sightedness (myopia) are also more susceptible to the development of glaucoma.

All patients over age 40 and particularly those at special risk need a regular examination for the presence of glaucoma. Detection of the earliest stages of the disease requires the use of special tools to measure pressure and the careful examination of the back of the eye.

Important Points In Treatment

When elevated pressure is found, it is treated even if there are no symptoms traceable to the increased pressure. It is best to begin

75

treatment before visual changes can be found. The changes in vision are not reversible.

Treatment can involve eyedrops (topical therapy), systemic drugs, or both. Either kind of therapy can produce side effects and beneficial effects. There is a need to document that the therapy is effective by repeated examination of the eye and its pressures. Therefore, glaucoma therapy is done under the care of an ophthalmologist.

Notify Our Office If

● If you experience acute eye pain.

Dry Eyes

Patient and Caregiver's Guide

 ## General Information

Dry eyes may be the consequence of decreased tear formation, the result of a slow blink rate, or both. Blinking, which is such an automatic function that few of us are aware of, spreads a thin film of tears over the eye. A slow blink rate may allow this film of tears to dry. Eye dryness results in a small but real change in visual acuity. Television may be a little less clear and crisp, and glare may be worse at night.

Elderly patients are more susceptible to dry eyes for several reasons. Changes that occur in the eye with aging may result in a decrease in the total output of tears. Many drugs, such as those used for the treatment of Parkinson's disease, glaucoma, depression, and gastrointestinal problems, can decrease the total volume of tears as a side effect. Problems that cause muscle weakness can lower the blink rate.

A number of diseases are associated with dry eyes. Chronic infections of the eye or the lids may be a cause. Neurologic changes following some strokes may lead to dry eye. Lack of vitamin A may cause this as well.

The environment may also contribute to the problem of dry eyes. Air conditioning lowers humidity. Prolonged residence in a dry, air-conditioned atmosphere can speed the drying rate and add to the problem of dry eyes. This may also occur during airplane travel. High-flying, pressurized, air-conditioned planes are notoriously low in humidity. The widespread use of dry forced-air heating in winter also leads to prolonged periods of low humidity and can make the problem of dry eyes worse. Elderly patients are particularly susceptible to these environmental conditions.

Most people are familiar with the gritty, irritating feeling of dry eyes. Often there is an associated infection, with the eyeball appearing red and with dilated blood vessels. In cases in which the cause of dry eyes is not readily apparent, it is possible for the ophthalmologist to conduct a test to evaluate tear production.

77

Important Points In Treatment

Your doctor will examine the eyes to discover whether any of the conditions associated with dry eye are a cause of the problem. There is a standard test that can be used to determine whether the eye is manufacturing an adequate volume of tears. Treatment of the underlying condition, if possible, is important to the management of dry eyes. The dry eye itself is most easily managed with the use of artificial tears. These are drops that may be put in the eye as needed to renew the tear film. You must be careful to keep the dropper tip clean. Eye drops come in small bottles intentionally to ensure that patients change to new, clean droppers regularly. Dirty droppers can lead to eye infections. Your ophthalmologist can advise you about the suitability of other slow-release preparations of artificial tears.

Notify Our Office If

- You have a persistent problem with glare that interferes with vision. Dry eyes lead to a small but real change in visual acuity. Television may be a little less clear and crisp, and glare may be worse at night.
- You experience red eyes or burning after starting a new medication. Several drugs produce dry eyes as a side effect. These include some but not all of the drugs used for the treatment of Parkinson's disease, anxiety, depression, diarrhea, irritable bowel syndrome, and heart arrhythmias.
- You have sudden onset of *redness* and *burning* in your eye. These symptoms can suggest eye infection. Dry eyes are most easily managed with the use of artificial tears, but you must be careful to keep the dropper tip clean. Dirty droppers lead to eye infections.

Sudden Visual Loss

Patient and Caregiver's Guide

General Information

A sudden loss of vision or partial loss of vision in one eye is an urgent warning sign of clogging of the blood vessels. This sort of change may involve the entire field of vision in one eye or it may affect only a part of the field of vision. A patient may experience the sensation of a curtain descending over one eye with a fading of vision. The term that physicians use for this condition is *amaurosis fugax*. A more common term is *transient monocular blindness* or *fleeting blindness* involving only one eye.

This occurs when the blood flow to the retina, which is the part of the eye that receives the light images, is temporarily cut off. Interruption of blood flow of no more than a few seconds will cause this sort of visual loss. If the interruption of blood flow continues, the loss of vision will become permanent.

Important Points In Treatment

The occurrence of transient monocular blindness is an important warning sign of the possibility of a stroke. When it occurs it should not be ignored. *The problem should be brought to the attention of your physician immediately*. It cannot wait for your next scheduled visit to your physician or eye doctor.

Notify Our Office If

- You develop a sudden change in vision, particularly if it involves only one eye.
- If the visual loss is only transient and normal vision promptly returns.
- You develop a sudden change in vision that is not transient or momentary and that involves only one eye. Call a doctor or visit an emergency room.

Retinal Tears and Retinal Detachment

Patient and Caregiver's Guide

General Information

The specialized layer in the back of the eye receives the image and transmits it to the brain. Under certain circumstances, this layer can be torn and, at times, separate from the back of the eye. When this occurs vision will deteriorate, and areas of blindness, in what are called the *visual fields,* may occur. Rapid treatment can arrest the progression of the tear or separation and preserve vision. It is the separation of the retina, the retinal detachment, that causes loss of vision. Failure to treat this may result in complete blindness in the affected eye.

Retinal tears may be asymptomatic, but they can also lead to retinal detachment and blindness. Even though most tears do not lead to blindness they are usually treated to stabilize them. Another form of retinal detachment occurs when fluid accumulates between layers, causing them to separate. Injury to the eye may also be associated with retinal detachment.

Retinal detachments occur in individuals with diabetic changes in their eye. Individuals with substantial degrees of nearsightedness also seem predisposed to the development of tears and/or detachment. Retinal detachment can also be a complication of cataract surgery.

Important Points In Treatment

Most important is the rapid diagnosis that will permit the initiation of treatment. Diagnosis is usually made by an ophthalmologist and frequently a retinal specialist. Anyone experiencing a sudden change in vision, the sudden development of floaters, or an awareness of flashes of light occurring spontaneously should contact an ophthalmologist for an immediate appointment.

Patients with a known predisposition for the development of retinal tears or retinal detachment should have regular examinations of their eyes to determine the possible presence of an asymptomatic tear. These could include individuals with diabetes and individuals with nearsightedness.

Notify Our Office If

- You notice a sudden change in vision.
- You experience an increase in the number of floaters in your eye.
- You begin to see spontaneous flashes of light.

Ptosis (Drooping of the Eyelid)

Patient and Caregiver's Guide

General Information

Drooping of one or both of the eyelids is called *ptosis* (pronounced *toe-sis*) or *blepharoptosis*. It may involve one or both eyes. There are many causes of a drooping eyelid, some of which are particularly common in the elderly. Often the drooping comes on very gradually, and the patient is not aware of the change.

Ptosis, or drooping eyelid, in the elderly is usually a result of a mechanical change in the support of the eyelid. Gradual stretching of the skin with age will permit the lid to droop. Eye infections, trauma, or surgery to the eye may accelerate these changes. The tendon that attaches to the muscle that opens the eyelid may become stretched either with age or because of these circumstances. Other diseases can also cause drooping eyelids.

Important Points In Treatment

Drooping eyelids alone rarely cause visual impairment. The physician's concern is with the possible underlying diseases that can cause the droop and may themselves require treatment. Patients are often bothered by the cosmetic appearance of the drooping lids. In the absence of underlying disease, little—other than plastic surgery—can be done to reverse the drooping lid.

Notify Our Office If

- You become aware of drooping eyelids.

Hearing Loss (Presbycusis)

Patient and Caregiver's Guide

General Information

Hearing loss has many possible causes. If there is interference in the ear itself, the hearing loss is called *conductive deafness*. The other major cause of hearing loss, *neural hearing deafness* (nerve deafness), is interference with the transmission from the ear to the brain. Both types of hearing loss occur with increased frequency in elderly patients. Presbycusis is the principal cause of the hearing loss of aging. It is a neural form of hearing loss. The occurrence and severity of the hearing loss are highly variable from patient to patient. High blood pressure, heredity, and a history of exposure to noise are all important factors in determining how severe and how progressive the hearing loss will be.

Prolonged exposure to loud noises may impair the ability to hear selective frequencies and sounds. Hearing protection during exposure to loud noises can forestall this change.

Usually the hearing loss involves higher-pitched sounds, but it is progressive in that it gradually involves sounds of lower pitch. At first, the ability to hear speech is intact, but eventually the loss progresses, and some speech sounds can no longer be heard.

Physicians recognize four different causes or types of presbycusis. Your physician will use audiometry (a hearing test) to begin the evaluation of your hearing loss.

Important Points In Treatment

The most important feature in the management of hearing loss is recognizing that a loss has occurred. Most of the management consists of a mix of supplementing the loss with properly selected, properly fitted hearing aids, and accommodating for the loss with appropriate environmental adjustments.

A hearing aid can compensate for some kinds of hearing loss. The hearing aid's performance must be matched with the kind of

83

hearing defect to provide any benefit at all. Even carefully selected and properly fitted hearing aids require a period of training on the part of the wearer to be effective. The patient must learn to use the hearing aid. It is unlikely that the hearing aid will completely restore normal hearing, and it is this new kind of hearing that the patient must learn in order to appreciate its benefit. A hearing aid is not an instant solution for a hearing defect.

Hearing aids require maintenance to function optimally. Changing tiny batteries can be difficult for elderly patients.

Care with communication can supplement the benefits of a hearing aid or compensate when a hearing aid is ineffective.

A few simple rules will make communicating with the hearing-impaired person easier:

- Eliminate as much of the background noise as is reasonably possible.
- The speaker should face the hearing-impaired person. Do not shout from another room or speak to the hearing-impaired person's back.
- Arrange the positioning and the lighting so that the hearing-impaired person can see the face of the speaker. Even without a knowledge of lip reading, a listener gets many clues from watching the speaker speak.
- Ask the speaker to speak distinctly. Slow speech is not particularly helpful. Do not shout.

Notify Our Office If

- You have a problem understanding conversation. The most important feature in the management of hearing loss is recognizing that the loss has occurred.

Hearing Aids

Patient and Caregiver's Guide

General Information

Almost all hearing impairments, short of total deafness, can be helped with a properly fitted hearing aid. Proper fitting requires a careful examination of the current level of hearing by performing an audiogram. This will identify the areas of the sound spectrum that the patient is unable to hear properly. This permits the audiologist to select the appropriate hearing aid to match the individual hearing defects of a specific patient.

Hearing aids are expensive and are only rarely covered by health insurance. For this reason, the patient is customarily offered a trial period, during which he or she is able to use the hearing aid to see whether it is a suitable solution. There are many different kinds of hearing aids, some equipped with sophisticated electronics that permit subtle adjustments of sound quality. Most hearing aids are now small enough to be contained within the ear and many within the ear canal itself.

In addition to hearing aids, there are other amplifying devices that can be used to improve the hearing for partially deaf individuals. There are telephones equipped with amplification that can greatly improve telephone communication for the hearing-impaired. Many hearing aids must be removed when using a telephone. In addition, there are devices that can be attached to radios, television sets, and sound systems that permit the amplified sound to be sent directly to headphones with a wireless connection. Systems of this sort are frequently available in theaters and churches.

Important Points In Treatment

A hearing aid, even if properly fitted, will rarely be able to restore normal hearing. The general rule of thumb is that the hearing loss will be cut in half. This will permit a restoration of communication, but it may not completely restore the ability to enjoy music.

If the hearing loss is approximately equal in each ear, the most effective restoration will involve fitting a hearing aid in each ear. This facilitates the ability to recognize the direction that sounds are coming from and usually provides better understanding of conversation. If there are substantial differences in the hearing loss between the two ears, it may not be possible to use two hearing aids.

Although hearing aids are sturdy devices, they must be handled with care, particularly in environments in which they might be dropped into water. This can cause irretrievable damage to the electronics. They should not be worn in the shower, and, in fact, it is prudent to not change or remove the hearing aid in the bathroom.

Notify Our Office If

- You find that you are experiencing hearing difficulties.

Dizziness (Vertigo)

Patient and Caregiver's Guide

General Information

Dizziness is described by some individuals as a feeling of faintness and by others as a feeling of rotary motion, when no rotary motion is actually occurring. The feeling of rotary motion is also called *vertigo*. Sometimes a dizzy person feels that he or she is revolving, whereas another sees the environment revolving around him or her. Other associated phenomena, such as light-headedness, may be harder to describe. Many people call this vertigo. Nausea and vomiting may accompany dizziness. This is a common association with motion sickness (sea sickness). Fainting and blackouts are also associated in some patients. Most dizziness reflects some problem with the inner ear, which is the vestibular apparatus that functions to keep humans balanced and upright. Dizziness is also occasionally due to a problem in the brain.

Historic details are of immense help to your physician in the evaluation of dizziness. Keep a few notes. Does the dizziness come on with changes in position? Is it present at rest? In bed? With exercise? While driving or in motion in another vehicle? Is there nausea or vomiting? Are there blackouts or weakness? Is there a position or an activity that relieves the dizziness?

Important Points In Treatment

Dizziness has many possible causes, and for each there is a specific kind of treatment. Careful, accurate diagnosis is essential to establish the cause and to select the appropriate management. Acute attacks of dizziness can be severe enough to be completely incapacitating. Be careful to prevent falls and possible injury. Stairs may be treacherous. Driving is a particular hazard.

Notify Our Office If

- You have dizziness. Causes of dizziness may be as trivial as a ride on a merry-go-round or as serious as a brain tumor. Report to your physician if dizziness occurs without a reasonable explanation.

Tinnitus

Patient and Caregiver's Guide

General Information

Tinnitus is the hearing of sounds, either in one or in both ears, that are not occurring in the environment. It is often but not invariably associated with hearing loss. Each individual may describe the sounds that he or she hears differently. Bells, ringing, whistling, and hissing are common descriptions.

Tinnitus has many possible causes. Some are local and can be trivial and temporary, such as blockage of the ear canal with wax. There are many individuals who have tinnitus without any explanation that can be found. On occasion this may be perceived as being so loud that it interferes with concentration during the day and restful sleep at night. Many causes involve other serious diseases. Tinnitus may be a reaction to a drug. Aspirin use is probably the most common cause of tinnitus at all ages.

Although tinnitus may occur at any age, elderly patients are particularly susceptible. Changes in the aging ear are sufficient to produce tinnitus in many people. Blood vessel changes that occur with aging may produce tinnitus. A blood vessel cause may be suspected if the sound is pulsating and, particularly, if it is in time with the heartbeat.

Important Points In Treatment

The treatment choices depend on the cause of the tinnitus. Evaluation by your physician to determine the cause is important for the treatment of the tinnitus. When tinnitus is associated with hearing loss, the use of a hearing aid often helps suppress the tinnitus. Tinnitus may be worsened by stress or tension. If tinnitus is a particular problem for you at night and interferes with falling asleep, the addition of soft background music with a timed clock radio or with a white noise or sound generator may help.

Notify Our Office If

- You experience ringing in the ears. Evaluation is important because of the common association of tinnitus with serious problems.

Otitis Externa (Swimmer's Ear)

Patient and Caregiver's Guide

General Information

Swimmer's ear is caused by inflammation in the external ear canal. It is usually caused by a bacterial or fungal infection that results when moisture is retained in the ear canal. Because the ear canal has little or no surrounding fat and is close to cartilage and bone, any swelling that occurs with the inflammation will cause pain in the ear. There may also be itching in the ear canal, and, if the swelling is sufficient to cause the canal to shut, there will be hearing loss as well.

Another cause of otitis externa may be trauma to the ear canal. Because the skin layer is thin and backed by bone or cartilage, it is easily injured if one uses undue force or a sharp object when attempting to remove ear wax.

Important Points in Management

Generally your physician will treat swimmer's ear by removing any obstruction and applying antibacterial agents or antibiotics directly into the ear canal. Removal of obstructions from the ear canal can be a delicate process and may require referral to an ear, nose, and throat specialist.

During the period of treatment the ear canal must be kept dry. With severe infections oral or injected antibiotics may be required. If the canal is swollen, the doctor may have to place a wick in the canal to promote drainage and to permit medicines to get into the canal.

Notify Our Office If

- You develop an itchy ear canal or a painful ear.

Otitis Media (Ear Infection)

Patient and Caregiver's Guide

General Information

Otitis media is an infection of the middle ear. It is very common in children but can also occur in adults. The chamber of the middle ear is connected to the outside through a hollow tube, the eustachian tube, that leads down to the throat. Air may enter or leave through this tube to keep the pressure in the middle ear equal to the outside pressure. This is important because of the pressure changes that occur when one changes altitude, as in a tall building elevator or in an airplane.

Colds (upper respiratory tract infection) and an airplane trips are the common causes of dysfunction of the eustachian tube, although there are many other less-common causes. When this tube is not working properly, an accumulation of fluid may occur in the middle ear. If this becomes infected, it is called *otitis media*. Infection here causes pain in the ear, vertigo (dizziness), and drainage from the ear; it may interfere with hearing. The infection may also cause fever.

Important Points In Treatment

The doctor can usually make the diagnosis of otitis media by looking into the ear canal and inspecting the eardrum. Treatment usually requires antibiotics and may require drainage of the middle ear infection through a hole made in the eardrum.

When the changes are chronic, the fluid behind the eardrum may not drain readily, and it may be necessary to insert tubes into the middle ear space through the eardrum. Chronic infections, if not treated promptly, may lead to hearing loss. It is also possible for hard lumps called *cholesteatomas* to form.

Call Our Office If

- You develop pain in the ear, particularly if you also have a fever.
- You develop drainage from the ear.
- You develop pain in the ear that is associated with hearing loss or tinnitus (ringing in the ears).

Taste

General Information

The sensations associated with taste are susceptible to changes with aging. These changes in taste may cause a change in your desire to eat. This, in turn, may affect your nutrition. Your taste sensations may disappear. Physicians call this *ageusia*. It is much less common than partial loss of taste, called *hypogeusia,* or a change in taste sensation, called *dysgeusia.*

These changes can be entirely caused by the aging process. They are often made worse or occur more quickly in patients taking a wide variety of drugs. A number of medical conditions are also associated with changes in taste sensation. Hence, for many reasons, in the elderly, taste sensations become less intense. This, in turn, leads to malnutrition and progressive weight loss. Weight loss in the elderly may progress to wasting, which directly affects one's health and quality of life.

Important Points In Treatment

Blunting of the sensation of taste makes it difficult for the elderly to be stimulated by food. This stimulation is important for triggering the digestive process. This coupled with the decrease in palatability leads to poor nutrition. Your doctor will review your medical history, particularly your medication history. This is an attempt to find an association with the reduction in the sense of taste that can be changed or corrected to restore some of the lost sense. When the change is a result of aging rather than drugs or disease, it may not be reversible.

Consider an experiment with condiments and flavors that intensify the taste of foods. Try a diet that reaches beyond the blunted taste threshold. Bland foods, which are often the traditional fare of the elderly, may do more nutritional harm than good.

For diabetic patients, the loss of the ability to taste or the raising of the threshold for sweet taste may lead to the excessive ingestion of sugar. In patients on a salt-restricted diet, the raising of the threshold for the taste of salt can lead to excessive salt ingestion.

Notify Our Office If

- You experience a change in the taste of foods.
- You have a change in your sense of taste.
- You develop progressive or unexplained weight loss.

Smell

General Information

The sensation of odor or sense of smell is susceptible to change with aging. Physicians call an absence of the sense of smell *anosmia*. This is less common as a result of aging than is impairment of the sense of smell, which physicians call *hyposmia*. Sometimes the ability to smell becomes distorted. Physicians call this *dysosmia*. Any of these changes affect the ability of a person to appreciate odors in the environment. When this happens, it changes the ability to appreciate food and other elements of the environment.

Loss of smell (and taste) is associated with a decrease in appetite. This, in turn, leads to malnutrition and progressive weight loss. Weight loss in the elderly may progress to wasting, which directly affects health and the quality of life.

Important Points In Treatment

Your doctor will review your medical history, particularly your medication history. This is an attempt to find an association with the reduction in the sense of smell that can be changed or corrected to restore some of the lost sense. When the change is a result of aging rather than drugs or disease it may not be reversible.

An additional approach to treatment is to use flavor enhancers in food preparation. These are natural essences that augment natural odors in food. They are not spices, although some spices can also be used to enhance the odor of prepared foods.

It helps to place a variety of foods on the plate. When only a single food is offered, it is possible for the odor of that food to tire the nose and lose much of its effect. When there is a variety of foods on the plate, one has less fatigue of the nose.

Notify Our Office If

- You have a change in your sense of smell.
- You develop progressive or unexplained weight loss.

CHAPTER 7

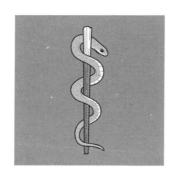
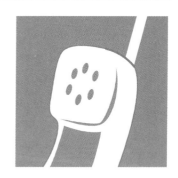

Incontinence

Incontinence (General)

Patient and Caregiver's Guide

General Information

Urinary incontinence (inability to hold the urine) is often part of the aging process. After age 65, about 10% of men and 20% of women have some incontinence. Incontinence is a severe problem in less than 5%. Often incontinence is temporary. Listed below are eight general causes of incontinence.

1. *Infection.* Sometimes bladder infection alone may cause sufficient discomfort that results in loss of bladder control. At other times, infection is just one problem, among others, that together result in incontinence.

2. *Weakening of the muscle that supports the bladder.* Weakening of the muscle that supports the bladder results in stress incontinence, which is the loss of small amounts of urine during coughing or sneezing. It usually occurs in women. Mild stress incontinence responds to regular exercises that strengthen the muscles supporting the bladder. Severe stress incontinence requires surgery to correct the supporting muscles.

3. *Weakening of the muscle of the bladder itself.* Partial obstruction of the bladder outlet causes weakening of the bladder muscle itself. This muscle change in the bladder most often occurs in men who have an enlarged prostate. It also occurs with nervous system problems, such as stroke, Parkinson's disease, and dementia.

4. *Nerve disorder.* Nerve disorders may cause loss of sensation in the bladder or control of the bladder. When bladder tightening cannot be controlled, bladder emptying can occur at any time.

5. *Delirium.* The confusion and disorientation associated with delirium may cause the patient to experience urinary incontinence.

6. *Drugs.* Incontinence may be the side effect of a drug, or it may be a secondary effect of the desirable result of a drug's action. The administration of diuretics (water pills) to a patient with

fluid retention and edema or swelling may produce such a copious output of urine that the patient becomes incontinent.

7. *Other diseases.* Additional causes of incontinence may be other illnesses, such as heart disease or diabetes, which, if not well controlled, will cause a copious outflow of urine.

8. *Surgery and/or radiation treatment to pelvic structures.* Most commonly, prostate tumors in men and uterine and cervical tumors in women may produce incontinence as a side effect.

Important Points In Treatment

When you are experiencing incontinence, one way to limit dribbling or uncontrolled release of urine at nighttime is to adjust the timing of when you drink fluids. This does not mean to stop fluid intake, for this would cause dehydration and is considered dangerous; it simply means to drink fluids at certain times and to limit them at others. For instance, to minimize incontinence at night or before going on a trip, do not drink large quantities for 2 hours before bedtime or before an outing. You can drink small amounts to keep your mouth moist or if you have to take medication at a specific time (e.g., before bed).

If you are experiencing incontinence, make sure you have a clear path to the bathroom so that you can get there in a hurry from your bed at night. Alternatively, place a portable commode next to your bed so that it is right there when you need it.

Garments are available to protect you during episodes of incontinence (called continence garments), and pads are available to protect your furniture and bedding (called incontinence pads). If you carefully select garments that fit your needs, you will ensure that you can continue to lead an active social life without embarrassment or odor.

For men, a number of urine collection (drainage) appliances are available to control incontinence. Your physician may occasionally insert a catheter to aid in emptying the bladder. Catheters carry a risk of infection, however, and a catheter by itself may not be proper treatment of incontinence.

Notify Our Office If

- You have any evidence of infection. Patients with incontinence are susceptible to infection of the urinary tract. This infection can cause fever, chills, a burning sensation on urination, frequent urination, cloudy urine, or bloody urine. Sometimes with incontinence, you may have an infection of the urinary tract but may not have any of these symptoms.

- You have any change in your urinary habits. A change indicates that something is wrong, whether it is an infection, another illness, or a side effect of your medication.
- You have any evidence of blood in your urine.

Stress Incontinence
Patient and Caregiver's Guide

General Information

Urinary incontinence is the inability to control urination. It has many causes. The problem may originate with the bladder or with the urethra, which is the canal that leads the urine from the bladder to the outside of the body. Often incontinence is the result of other illnesses and is only temporary. Incontinence varies from occasional episodes to total loss of bladder control.

Stress incontinence is a problem in older women. In these women, small amounts of urine are lost when they sneeze, cough, or strain suddenly. This occurs because of increased pressure within the abdomen and the inability of the muscles to support the bladder during intervals of increased pressure or stress. The weakened muscles are a normal part of the aging process, but they usually do not weaken to the point of causing stress incontinence.

If your condition is mild, physical therapy can help by strengthening the muscles that support the bladder. You may not see results right away, but in a few months you should see results if you continue to exercise regularly. Sometimes your physician may prescribe some type of support device that is inserted vaginally, like a tampon or a pessary. In more severe cases, surgery may restore the weakened area so that the bladder can resist sudden straining, sneezing, or coughing without the unintentional release of urine.

Important Points In Treatment

If you have stress incontinence, your physician will carefully evaluate you to be sure that you have no infection of the urinary tract. You should have with you a list of all the medications you are currently taking. Include your over-the-counter (nonprescription) drugs as well as your prescription drugs. Drugs do not cause stress incontinence, but some cause the condition to get worse.

Exercises are often helpful, particularly Kegel's exercises. The goal of these exercises is to make you aware of and be in control of the muscles that are involved in urination. The best way to become aware of these muscles is to stop your urinary stream and then restart it voluntarily. Become familiar with the process of tightening, stopping urination, relaxing, and then starting urination with these muscles. Once you are familiar with these muscles, try tightening and relaxing them at other times (when not urinating). Do these exercises three times daily, starting with five sets (repetitions) of tightening and then relaxing the muscles at each session, for a total of 15 sets per day. Progress slowly up to 25 sets (repetitions) at each session, for a total of 75 sets per day.

Overweight patients will notice a decrease in the frequency of involuntary urination when they lose weight.

Notify Our Office If

- You have any evidence of a urinary tract infection. Any of the following symptoms may indicate that you have such an infection: burning sensation while urinating, frequent urination of small amounts, cloudy urine, bloody urine, fever, or chills.
- You experience a return of symptoms of stress incontinence. This is particularly important if symptoms return after you have had successful surgery to repair the bladder support area or after you have successfully completed your exercise therapy and have built up the muscles in that area. The return of symptoms could mean that you have an infection that needs treatment.

Incontinence and Prostatic Disease

Patient and Caregiver's Guide

General Information

As men get older, the prostate gland gets larger, a condition known as *benign prostatic hyperplasia*. Many men do not become incontinent even though they have an enlarged prostate. In some men, however, an enlarged prostate may cause problems because it can put pressure on the bladder, resulting in the frequent release of small quantities of urine. You may feel the need to urinate at night. You may also find it difficult to get your stream of urine started, and then you may find that your bladder is emptying very slowly. Sometimes the interference of the enlarged prostate with the bladder area causes minor incontinence, referred to as dribbling.

Malignant tumors may also develop in the prostate. Unfortunately, these tumors do not always produce symptoms.

Important Points In Treatment

Surgical removal of part of the enlarged prostate is the usual treatment for benign prostatic hyperplasia. An alternative, non-surgical treatment with drugs alone may be used at times when symptoms are mild.

After surgery, there may be a period of incontinence, but this should end sometime during the subsequent 6 months. An extremely small percentage of patients (1%) may continue to have mild dribbling when in an upright position. Continence garments and incontinence pads should offer a comfortable solution while you attempt to improve this condition by means of pelvic muscle exercises. Kegel's exercises are particularly helpful. The goal of these exercises is to make you aware of and be in control of the muscles that are involved in urination. The best way to become aware of these muscles is to stop your urinary stream and then restart it voluntarily. Become familiar with the process of tightening, stopping urination, relaxing, and then starting urination with these muscles. Once you are familiar with these muscles, try tightening and relaxing them at other times (when not urinating). Do these exercises three times daily, starting with five sets (repetitions) of tightening and then relaxing the muscles at each session, for a total of 15 sets per day. Progress slowly up to 25 sets (repetitions) each session, for a total of 75 sets per day.

Occasionally, surgery to correct benign prostatic hyperplasia affects potency, but, because the disease occurs at a time in life when sexual activity is decreasing anyway, it is not clear whether surgery is actually the cause of the decreased potency. Most patients experience little, if any, actual change in potency. This surgery occasionally causes retrograde ejaculation (emptying of ejaculate into the bladder rather than directly through the penis). Sterility does result but impotence does not.

Even though the removal of prostate tumors requires more extensive surgery, the postoperative effects are similar to those that occur after surgery for benign prostatic hyperplasia. The effects become more severe, however, if there is more extensive surgery for removal of the tumor.

 ## Notify Our Office If

- You have urinary incontinence.
- You must urinate frequently but with small volumes during the daytime or are awakened frequently from sleep to urinate.

Incontinence and Dementia

General Information

Dementia is a loss of intellectual function. Impaired mental status may sometimes result in the development of urinary incontinence. This happens because patients who lose their mental awareness may release their bladder contents when they feel the urge. The severity of the incontinence generally corresponds with the severity of the dementia.

Other complicating factors may occur. A number of the drugs used to treat the dementia may produce incontinence as a side effect. Infection of the urinary tract causes frequent urges to urinate and may be an underlying cause of the incontinence. Sometimes incontinence occurs because of nighttime confusion or wandering that prevents access to a toilet.

Important Points In Treatment

If you are caring for an incontinent person, you face a difficult challenge. Frequently incontinence becomes a reason to refer a patient to a nursing home. Your patience will be tested. Partial continence is possible in less-severely demented patients, which improves the quality of life of the caregiver as well as of the patient. The patient's physician will try to control the factors that may be causing the incontinence.

Geography

Your patient needs ready access to toilet facilities. The bedroom should have direct access to the bathroom, there should be a night-light in the bedroom, and a soft light should remain on in the bathroom. If the patient is unsteady physically, you can have grab bars and an elevated toilet seat installed. If you cannot make these bedroom and bathroom arrangements, a bedside commode is an effective substitute.

Fluid Management

You can partially control the patient's urinary output by controlling the times when the patient drinks fluids. For instance, you can minimize incontinence while the patient is sleeping by having the patient avoid drinking large amounts for 2 hours before bedtime. This does not mean fluid restriction, because adequate daily fluid intake is important for good health. Small amounts of fluid help to keep the mouth comfortably moist. In addition, the patient may have to take medication right before bedtime.

Nursing Aids

Special garments (continence garments) are available from commercial suppliers. Incontinence pads are also available to protect furniture and bedding. Careful selection of the right garment will allow the patient to have a comfortable social life without embarrassment, despite episodes of incontinence. The right garment and pad will also make your life as a caregiver easier and less frustrating.

For men, a number of urine collection (drainage) appliances are available to control incontinence. These also have a role in the care of demented men. The physician may occasionally insert a catheter to aid with the emptying of the bladder. Catheters carry a risk of infection, however, and a catheter by itself may not be proper treatment for incontinence.

Notify Our Office If

- The patient has any evidence of a urinary tract infection. Patients with incontinence are susceptible to infection of the urinary tract. Urinary tract infection can cause fever, chills, a burning sensation on urination, frequent urination, cloudy urine, or bloody urine. Sometimes with incontinence the patient may have an infection of the urinary tract but may not have any of these symptoms.
- The patient has any change in urinary habits. A change indicates that something is wrong, whether it is an infection, another illness, or a side effect of the patient's medication.
- The patient has any evidence of blood in the urine.

Fecal Incontinence

Patient and Caregiver's Guide

 ## General Information

Few things are as disturbing to patients and caregivers alike as an inability to control bowel movements and remain continent. It is not an aging change, but it is a problem that is associated with many age-related health problems. Because of the difficulties associated with providing nursing care for an incontinent patient, the development of this problem is often the underlying cause for nursing home placement. Patients thrive best in their own home environment; therefore, every effort should be made to restore continence or manage incontinence. Physicians divide incontinence into three varieties based on cause. The treatment varies with each of these causes.

1. Overflow incontinence occurs when a patient has suffered constipation, which permits the development of a fecal impaction. A fecal impaction is a hard mass of feces that collects just above the outlet and is too large to pass. The patient loses the ability to discriminate between gas, fluids, and feces, and therefore leakage occurs. Overflow incontinence is managed by removal of the impaction and prevention of its recurrence.

2. Anorectal incontinence occurs when there has been damage to the nerves that supply impulses to the rectum and anus. This causes the rectal sphincter (the muscle that keeps the anus closed) to weaken, and the anus may actually gape open. Exercise and retraining of these muscles may help to restore continence, but surgery is needed in some situations.

3. Neurologic incontinence occurs when there is central nervous system difficulty, such as stroke or dementia. Careful timing of meals and visits to the commode permit avoidance of an episode of incontinence. Occasionally laxatives or suppositories are used to adjust the timing of bowel movements. The use of drugs should be under the direction of a physician. The goal is to restore a normal pattern, not to adjust the timing of bowel movements to the convenience of a caregiver.

In some cases, retraining using a process called *biofeedback* may permit the restoration of continence and control. Biofeedback training is usually done in specialized centers and requires a course or interval of training to achieve maximum benefit.

Summary

- Patients thrive best in their own home environment; thus, every effort should be undertaken to restore or manage incontinence.
- Symptomatic incontinence occurs as a result of other intestinal tract diseases. These other problems are the focus of treatment, and their resolution often also resolves the incontinence.

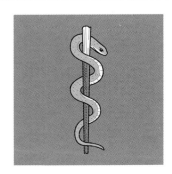
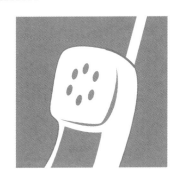

Gastrointestinal Problems

Dental Hygiene

Patient and Caregiver's Guide

General Information

Dental problems have a great impact on the quality of life. Besides the pain and discomfort associated with cavities (caries), the loss of teeth makes it difficult to chew food properly. This, in turn, may lead to poor nutrition. Prevention is always better than treatment. Prevention of caries, even in teeth that are already damaged, can slow or arrest further progression of tooth problems. Benefits of preventive care continue to accrue at any age.

Tooth Loss

Most of the traditional images of elderly people are of people without teeth. However, tooth loss, although not uncommon, is not an essential element of aging. Some teeth are lost to changes in the bones of the jaw. Osteoporosis may occur in the bones that support the teeth, and, when it does, these teeth are more vulnerable to loss. Many more teeth are lost to periodontal disease, or inflammation of the gums, which exposes the roots of the teeth and facilitates decay. Most teeth are lost to decay.

Tooth Decay

Most people are surprised to learn that cavities are a kind of infectious disease. When bits of food remain in the mouth, bacteria attack the sugars in the food and convert them into acids. These acids, in turn, erode the calcium that makes up the teeth.

Careful after-meal cleaning can remarkably reduce the occurrence of tooth decay. When it is not possible to brush after meals, chewing a stick of sugarless gum can help clean the teeth and remove the acids. Careful cleaning before bedtime is important as well. Overnight, the tiny amounts of calcium that were removed from the teeth during the day are replaced by calcium in the saliva.

Periodontal Disease

Periodontal disease is inflammation of the gums. This inflammation causes the gums to recede and exposes the roots of the teeth to possible decay. The roots of the teeth are much less resistant to the effects of acid. Periodontal disease is a major predisposition to tooth loss and decay.

Prevention of periodontal disease requires careful cleaning of the teeth and the areas between the teeth. Your dentist can best advise you concerning the selection of a cleaning method. Dental floss, tiny brushes for between the teeth, and water-jet cleaners are useful tools.

Important Points In Treatment

Regular visits to your dentist and dental hygienist permit cleaning the teeth of plaque that is not removed by simple brushing or flossing. Preventive dentistry is the best safeguard against tooth problems. Careful brushing after meals and before bed can also help.

Many people note that with aging they begin to develop a thick white coat on the tongue. This is most noticeable on rising in the morning. A bacterium that seems to be more common in the elderly causes this. It has been associated with the development of some forms of tooth decay. Tongue brushing can remove much of this coat. Coarse foods, such as toast, may also remove it. People who skip breakfast or have only a cup of coffee should consider tongue brushing at the time of tooth brushing as a regular part of their dental hygiene.

Gingivitis

Patient and Caregiver's Guide

General Information

Gingivitis is the most visible sign of periodontal disease. It is a disease of the supporting structures of the teeth. Gum disease, like dental caries (cavities), is not a necessary consequence of the aging process. However, any break in dental hygiene can permit gingivitis or dental caries to gain a foothold. With the passage of time, these problems accumulate, and thus there is an apparent increase in occurrence in elderly patients. Most tooth loss in elderly patients is a result of periodontal disease, not cavities.

Gingivitis, like dental caries, is a result of mouth bacteria infecting normal tissues. These bacteria form plaque that can cling to the teeth. If plaque is left and accumulates, it can irritate the gums, causing them to become inflamed. The inflamed gums bleed and swell. It is these bleeding and swollen gums that we recognize as gingivitis. If permitted to persist, it may lead to the loss of bone and ligamentous support for the teeth. In turn, the teeth may loosen and fall out.

Important Points In Treatment

The control and reversal of gingivitis and the associated periodontal disease are as important as the prevention of its occurrence.

Prevention rests with good dental hygiene. Regular brushing and flossing minimize the development of plaque. If disease or disability impairs cleaning and flossing, plaque accumulation and gingivitis may result.

Several diseases may cause or exacerbate gingivitis and the underlying periodontal disease. Diabetes, for example, can slow healing and prolong the inflammation and swelling, even after hygiene is restored. Some drugs can irritate gums directly or indirectly by causing dry mouth. A few drugs can simulate gingivitis by causing noninflammatory swelling of the gums. It is important to give your physician and your dentist a complete list of your prescription and nonprescription medications.

If you have trouble maintaining regular brushing and flossing, it is possible to control plaque buildup by using a plaque-dissolving mouthwash. These mouthwashes contain chlorhexidine. Some cause staining of plastic tooth restoration material, and the advice of your dentist is important in the selection of the proper mouthwash for you.

Flossing requires two-handed dexterity. The use of water-jet cleaners requires only one-handed dexterity. These cleaners are useful for maintaining oral hygiene in patients with arthritis, stroke, or other problems that limit two-handed dexterity. Your dentist can best advise you about the appropriateness of daily cleaning with water-jet cleaners. There are flossing tools available that will permit single-handed flossing. These require some dexterity to do a complete job, but they do offer a less-expensive alternative to water-jet cleaners.

Often an increase in the frequency of visits to your dental hygienist can compensate, in part, for any difficulties with cleaning that you might have.

Notify Our Office If

- You have sore or bleeding gums.

Dry Mouth

Patient and Caregiver's Guide

General Information

Excessive dryness of the mouth can cause difficulty with talking and swallowing and can irritate or exacerbate gum disease, which results in tooth loss. Dry mouth is not a result of the aging process, but it may be a consequence of diseases related to aging or the treatment of these diseases.

Patients who have trouble chewing and swallowing dry foods or who often need to drink while chewing a mouthful of food may be experiencing dry-mouth syndrome. Hoarseness and difficulty speaking at length may also be complaints. Oral ulcerations, furrowing of the mucous membranes, and dental caries (cavities) are later features. Saliva is important for the maintenance of proper mineralization of the teeth.

Dry mouth is a side effect of many drugs—so many drugs (more than 400) that it is hard to anticipate which ones will cause significant dry mouth in any given patient. Many of these medications are a part of the management of problems of aging, such as Parkinson's disease, depression, and hypertension. A few diseases, including infections and tumors, can cause dry mouth as well.

Important Points In Treatment

Management may include adjusting medications to lessen the drying effects in the mouth. Some medications may need to be maintained because they are essential components of the treatment of other serious diseases. Treatment of diseases that can cause drying can be helpful.

A few drugs can effectively stimulate salivary secretions without bothersome side effects. Salivary substitutes are of limited help. Careful dental hygiene, including regular, frequent cleaning, can help to prevent caries and tooth loss.

Notify Our Office If

- The patient has a problem with dryness of the mouth.
- The patient has any evidence of dry mouth. Caregivers should remember that, if general awareness is impaired by dementia, medications, stroke, or other problems, no external signs serve as a clue to the presence of the problem.

Swallowing Difficulties

Patient and Caregiver's Guide

General Information

With age, the esophagus—the swallowing tube that leads from the mouth to the stomach—undergoes changes that may make it difficult to swallow and may impair coordination. When the esophagus is functioning normally, swallowed food moves by a muscular wave, called a *peristaltic wave,* rapidly down from the throat to the stomach. In adults, even when they are hanging upside down, it takes, at most, 11 seconds for swallowed food to make the trip to the stomach.

Aging changes impair this smooth coordination. A peristaltic wave may no longer follow every swallow. When this happens, the patient is often, but not always, aware of difficulty swallowing. Patients describe a feeling of food sticking somewhere down in the chest. Usually this sticking occurs with liquids as well as solids. It is often painless, but chest discomfort can occur. A spasm (a sort of charley horse) that involves the muscles in the esophagus has occurred. This slows the bolus of food, which actually does stick for a time instead of progressing smoothly down into the stomach.

Difficulties with a dry mouth may also present to some patients as difficulty swallowing. Dry mouth is common in the elderly. It has many possible causes. Some medications may cause dry mouth.

Important Points In Treatment

Treatment of esophageal spasm includes the use of drugs to decrease inflammation and to prevent reflux into the esophagus. Medication can also be given to relax or prevent a spasm in the esophageal muscle. Rarely, tight areas in the esophagus may need stretching, and, even more rarely, surgery is necessary.

If the difficulty is primarily because of a dry mouth, taking fluids with solid food may help the swallowing process.

Notify Our Office If

- You have any difficulty swallowing food or liquids.

Heartburn

General Information

Heartburn is a common problem. One fifth of adults in the United States have occasional heartburn, and 10% suffer daily attacks. With aging, changes occur in the ability of the esophagus, the swallowing tube that leads from the mouth to the stomach, to work smoothly. There is an associated increase in the occurrence of heartburn as one grows older.

The symptom of heartburn is usually a warm or burning feeling in the middle of the front of the chest. Bending, straining, or stooping often causes heartburn, and it is frequently worse when one lies down. Food or drink can relieve the burning sensation, as does the use of an antacid preparation. Such relief is temporary, because the problem is recurrent. Often particular foods cause heartburn. Icing on rolls or cake, orange juice, hot (spicy) foods, and hot dogs are common causes. Any individual may have a particular food that brings on the problem, although it may not be the same food that bothers other sufferers. A few patients with severe heartburn experience the regurgitation of food and acid into the mouth and throat. Sometimes they are aware of this only as a bitter taste in the mouth on awakening in the morning. On other occasions it is very apparent, producing irritation with coughing and choking.

Nighttime regurgitation while asleep can occur and occasionally permits acid or food to get into the windpipe. This can cause hoarseness and cough that on occasion is the only complaint related to the reflux. In some individuals this provokes wheezing and shortness of breath resembling asthmatic attacks. Acid coming up into the mouth at night may be the cause of erosion of the teeth. These complications may occur without the occurrence of heartburn.

Important Points In Treatment

If there is evidence of reflux with inflammation of the esophagus, treatment is undertaken to prevent the reflux and to heal the esophagus. Treatment may involve reducing the amount of acid available for reflux or reducing the reflux itself and frequently involves a combination of drugs to achieve both ends.

Commonly treatment is with medications to decrease acid secretion by the stomach. It is also possible to use antacids to neutralize the acid secretion. Special antacids taken after meals can mechanically prevent the reflux of acid and food and neutralize the acid. Other drugs can strengthen the muscle at the end of the esophagus that keeps the esophagus closed and mechanically prevents reflux from occurring.

Besides using these medicines, you can take several measures to prevent reflux. Reflux occurs more easily when you are lying flat than when sitting or standing. Elevation of the head of your bed on several bricks or elevation of the head of your mattress with a foam wedge can help you take advantage of gravity in the prevention of reflux. Propping up your head on several pillows is usually not helpful because it can still permit pooling of acid at the lower end of the esophagus at the point where one usually bends when elevating the head with a pillow. It is far better to try to raise the entire mattress on a slant to obtain the benefits of gravity.

An increase of pressure within the abdomen causes reflux. To reduce this, you should avoid tight-fitting or elastic garments and girdles or corsets. Bending over also increases pressure in the abdomen and adds the negative effect of gravity in causing reflux. This is particularly true if you bend over to pick up a heavy object. It is wiser to stoop down rather than to bend over when picking up something from the floor.

A full stomach refluxes more easily than an empty one. Avoid eating and drinking for at least 2 hours (3 would be better) before bedtime or before taking a nap lying down. Avoid foods that you know by experience promote reflux.

Complications may occur if reflux recurs for a long time without treatment. The acid refluxing into the esophagus may cause inflammation, producing an ulcer with or without bleeding. When the inflammation is severe, particularly with ulcerations, scarring may occur as the esophagus heals. Besides this, the irritation caused by the inflammation in the esophagus may make it clamp down in a muscle spasm that causes difficulty swallowing. If you have difficulty swallowing foods, report this to your physician. He or she will do an evaluation to find out whether scarring has occurred or whether it is simple muscular spasm from irritation that is causing the difficulty. This will permit a selection of the appropriate therapy to relieve your swallowing difficulties.

Notify Our Office If

- You have difficulty swallowing food.
- You experience persistent heartburn.
- You experience unexplained hoarseness.
- You have bouts of wheezing or asthma, particularly at night.
- Your dentist informs you that you are developing dental erosions.

Hiatal Hernia

Patient and Caregiver's Guide

General Information

A hiatal hernia occurs when the stomach protrudes through the opening in the diaphragm. It is a very common finding and occurs in approximately half the adult population of the United States. There are two types of hiatal hernia. The most common form is a sliding hiatal hernia. Far less common is a variety called a *paraesophageal hiatal hernia*. The paraesophageal variety may be associated with complications, such as bleeding. This type of hiatal hernia is not particularly a problem of elderly patients.

Sliding hiatal hernia does seem to occur with increasing frequency in elderly patients. The hernia itself only rarely causes a health problem, and then only if it is very large. Sliding hiatal hernia occurs with several other medical problems. Reflux of acid into the esophagus is common with a sliding hiatal hernia. Reflux produces heartburn and can cause scarring in the esophagus. These associated problems may require special diagnosis and treatment, and these problems, not the hiatal hernia, are the focus of your physician's attention.

Important Points In Treatment

The treatment of the symptoms caused by hiatal hernia involves the prevention of reflux of acid from the stomach into the esophagus. The following changes will reduce the occurrence of reflux:

1. Elevate the head of your bed. Use blocks or bricks under the head end of the bed. Simply propping your head up on pillows is not effective. A foam wedge made to be placed under the mattress can be used if you cannot elevate the head of your bed.
2. Do not eat or drink for at least 2 hours (3 would be better) before going to bed. If the stomach is nearly empty when you go to bed, there is little acid to reflux into the esophagus.
3. Do not wear tight, elastic, or restricting garments. Any binding that raises the pressure inside the abdominal cavity promotes reflux.

4. Stoop rather than bend over to pick up objects from the floor. This decreases the chance for reflux to occur.

Besides following these measures, you may be given medication by your physician, who may select from several medications that can decrease the acid production in the stomach, neutralize the acid, or strengthen the muscle in the lower esophagus to prevent reflux.

Notify Our Office If

- You experience frequent, persistent heartburn.
- You experience regurgitation of food into your mouth.
- You awaken with a bitter taste in your mouth and/or hoarseness.

Aspirin, NSAIDs, and Stomach Irritation

Patient and Caregiver's Guide

General Information

Effective treatment of inflammatory disease, such as rheumatoid arthritis, often includes the use of anti-inflammatory drugs. Aspirin and aspirin-like drugs, which are commonly called *non-steroidal* anti-inflammatory drugs, or NSAIDs, are among the mainstays of treatment of these inflammatory diseases.

The benefits of these drugs, the control of pain and the restoration of function in affected joints, must balance the possibility that gastrointestinal or other side effects may occur. NSAIDs can cause inflammation of the stomach, which, in turn, may lead to bleeding from the stomach with or without the occurrence of ulcers. Ulcerations without bleeding may occur as well. Some NSAIDs may also cause diarrhea and may affect the function of the kidneys. In a few people, aspirin causes attacks of asthma.

Not all people are equally susceptible to the effect of NSAIDs on the stomach. There are individuals with "cast-iron stomachs," people who are unusually sensitive, and all gradations in between.

Differences also exist among the various NSAIDs and their ability to cause irritation in the stomach. Some individuals may be more tolerant of one drug than another. Some newer drugs, COX-2 inhibitors, seem to have a substantially smaller, if any, effect on the stomach. Your physician needs your help to identify the drug and the dosage that is best suited for you.

Important Points In Treatment

Certain measures should be taken to reduce the harmful side effects of these drugs on the stomach. Anti-inflammatory drugs, like most medications, should be taken on a regular, scheduled basis. Generally, the effects of these drugs on the stomach are worse, if you take the drug when the stomach is empty. When possible, take doses with a meal. Food is a natural protection against stomach irritants. If a drug dose does not fall at a mealtime, a simple snack offers some protection. This snack may be no more than crackers and a glass of water. If even a snack is not permissible, a dose of an antacid preparation taken simultaneously may offer some beneficial protection to the stomach.

NSAIDs should be taken with adequate water or other beverages to ensure that the pills move into the stomach and do not remain stuck in the esophagus. Adequate fluid ensures that disintegrating tablets are diluted. Concentrated solutions of the drug result from taking only a swallow or two of water and may be more irritating than the diluted solutions that would occur by swallowing the pill with a full glass of water. Drink a full glass of water with each pill, or even two glasses, if possible.

If your physician prescribes NSAIDs and you have a known sensitivity to irritant side effects, or if high doses are necessary, your physician may suggest treatment with an additional drug to help protect the stomach.

Protective drug choices include preparations that suppress acid production or preparations that add a protective layer or coating to the stomach lining. Your physician will help you select the best drug. Interactions between these and other drugs can occur, so the choice varies with your total treatment program.

Complications

The side effects of NSAIDs may include gastritis, peptic ulceration, or both. Small amounts of bleeding from the stomach may occur with either problem, and, occasionally, major bleeding may result. Usually, patients with gastritis or an ulcer experience discomfort in the pit of the stomach. This may be felt as a burning or an ache, as a hunger pang, or, less commonly, as a sharp pain. This pain usually occurs in the center of the upper stomach but may occasionally occur in the sides or the back. Many patients are somewhat insensitive to discomfort and may have real inflammation in the stomach without feeling any symptoms at all. Your physician may request periodic checks of your blood count or tests for hidden (occult) blood in your stool. These tests are done to ensure that a problem is not missed in an unusually stoic patient.

Besides pain in the stomach, heartburn is also a possible presentation of stomach irritation. Heartburn is a very common problem; however, if its character changes by increasing in frequency, severity, or duration, notify your physician. Bleeding, although it often occurs, may be a concealed symptom. Occasionally a patient will vomit blood or pass fresh blood or maroon-colored blood in the stool. More often, altered blood in the stool is black and tarry. Your physician should be alerted immediately if any of these changes occur.

Notify Our Office If

- You have any evidence of bleeding from the gastrointestinal tract. The side effects of NSAIDs may include gastritis, peptic ulceration, or both. Small amounts of bleeding occur with either problem, and, occasionally, major bleeding may result.

Helicobacter Pylori Infection (Gastritis)

Patient and Caregiver's Guide

General Information

A great deal of public and scientific interest has been generated in a recently discovered infection that occurs in the stomach. Usually the acid in the stomach keeps this organ free of infections. However, one bacterium, *Helicobacter pylori,* has evolved a mechanism to tolerate this harsh environment.

When this organism first infects the stomach, it produces a brief interval of stomach upset. There may be nausea and vomiting, hunger pangs, and abdominal cramps. It is one of many causes of "intestinal flu" and, as such, passes unremarkably as one of the burdens that we all must bear.

However, unlike other infections that cause stomach upset, when the acute, early symptoms pass, this infection does not go away. It becomes a chronic or long-lasting infection in almost everyone it infects. Usually this chronic infection causes no complaints or symptoms; however, the chronic infection will, in some people, lead to the later development of stomach and duodenal ulcers. After very long intervals, probably decades, it may be a factor in the development of some stomach tumors.

Usually your physician will treat *H. pylori* infection, if it is present. Unlike many other infections, it does not require urgent or immediate treatment. Your physician needs to consider your other health problems and medications to decide the best time to treat this infection. The complications caused by chronic infection with the *H. pylori* organism require other treatment. Treatment of the chronic infection may wait until more pressing problems are under control.

Important Points In Treatment

Infection with the *H. pylori* organism is not difficult to treat, but its treatment does call for three or sometimes four drugs. Even the best treatment has a 10% failure rate, and retreatment is required for some patients. The drugs commonly used include the following:

- *Omeprazole (Prilosec), esomeprazole (Nexium), pantoprazole (Protonix), rabeprazole (Aciphex), or lansoprazole (Prevacid).* This medicine suppresses acid in the stomach. The *H. pylori* organism weakens in the absence of acid and is more susceptible to other drugs.
- *Ranitidine (Zantac), nizatidine (Axid), or famotidine (Pepcid).* This medicine also suppresses acid in the stomach. The *H. pylori* organism weakens in the absence of acid and is more susceptible to other drugs.
- *Amoxicillin.* This antibiotic is a special kind of penicillin.
- *Clarithromycin.* This antibiotic is highly effective against *H. pylori*.
- *Biaxin.* This is another kind of antibiotic.
- *Metronidazole (Flagyl).* This medication is an effective treatment, but it has side effects, if you drink alcohol while taking it.
- *Bismuth (Pepto-Bismol).* Bismuth is an excellent drug for infection with *H. pylori*. The only readily available source of bismuth in the United States is Pepto-Bismol. Bismuth will change stool color to black.

Notify Our Office If

- You must interrupt your treatment for more than a single dose of medication.

Treatment of *Helicobacter Pylori* Infection

Patient and Caregiver's Guide

General Information

Infection in the stomach with *H. pylori* will cause gastritis and may lead to the development of peptic ulcers and, in some cases, cancers of the stomach. For this reason, when this infection is found, it is usually treated.

The treatment of this infection usually involves the use of two antibiotics plus a drug to suppress the acid in the stomach. Treatment takes from 10 to 14 days. The success rate of treating this infection is usually in excess of 90%. There are several things that you can do to be sure that you received the maximum benefit from the treatment.

H. pylori lives in the mucous that lines the stomach wall. It does not infect the stomach wall by entering the cells, and it does not become a systemic infection in the body. The antibiotics used to treat it are effective while they are in the stomach. This sort of treatment is called *topical* treatment. In addition, this organism seems to be more susceptible to treatment if gastric acid has been suppressed during the time that the bacteria is exposed to the antibiotic. This means that the timing of the various medications and what you take with them, or do not take with them, in the form of food and drink, may have an effect on how successful they are for eradicating the organism.

The medications are usually given two times daily. These are all oral medications that are taken by mouth. The acid-suppressing drug should be taken on an empty stomach before breakfast in the morning and before bedtime. The evening dose should come at least 3 hours after the last meal. One half hour after the acid-suppressing medication is taken, the antibiotics should be taken. At the time the antibiotics are taken, you should have something to eat or drink that would ordinarily stimulate the stomach to

131

produce acid. It takes only a small meal or a snack to do this. Drinking coffee or tea or a beverage containing caffeine is also helpful in stimulating the stomach to get the maximum reduction of the gastric acid and the maximum effect from the antibiotic preparation. There should be an adequate volume of fluid to permit the antibiotics to dissolve in the stomach so that they may penetrate the mucous layer and reach the infecting organism. The volume should not be so large that it dilutes the concentration of the antibiotic in the stomach. Eight to twelve ounces of fluid is most suitable.

It is important to adhere as rigorously as possible to this regimen. Skipping or missing a dose of the treatment may markedly reduce the success of the treatment. It often requires a brief adjustment in lifestyle and some planning during the 2 weeks of therapy to ensure that it may be successfully completed. Therapy should be delayed if you are aware that your upcoming schedule will make it difficult to follow this program.

Proton Pump Inhibitors

Patient and Caregiver's Guide ▪ ▪ ▪

General Information

Proton pump on inhibitors are powerful drugs that inhibit the production of acid by the stomach. They are commonly used in the treatment of gastroesophageal reflux disease (GERD), peptic ulcer disease, and infection in the stomach with *Helicobacter pylori*. Many patients will find that they must remain on this medication for long intervals of time. To obtain the maximum effect of this drug, one must pay particular attention to timing when it is taken.

At the present time in the United States, five different proton pump inhibitors are available as prescription medications. These include Omeprazole (Prilosec), esomeprazole (Nexium), pantoprazole (Protonix), rabeprazole (Aciphex), and lansoprazole (Prevacid). In addition, one of these, omeprazole (Prilosec), is available without prescription as an over-the-counter medication.

This drug should be taken on an empty stomach. It should be taken 30 to 60 minutes before the meal. The tablets or the tiny pills inside the capsules should not be ground or chewed. They must remain intact to protect the drugs from being prematurely activated by the acid in the stomach. The medication must pass through the stomach intact and into the small intestine. The pills are designed to disintegrate in the small intestine to permit the drug to be absorbed into the blood. The circulation then carries the medication throughout the body. It will circulate for 1.5 hours on average before it is metabolized and gone.

Some of the drug is carried to the wall of the stomach to the cells that manufacture the stomach acid. When the cells begin to manufacture acid, which occurs when you eat a meal, the drug becomes activated and turns the acid-producing mechanism off. No further acid will be produced until the stomach manufactures additional acid-producing enzymes.

The timing of taking the medication 30 to 60 minutes before eating a meal permits the maximum effect of the medication in the inhibiting of the production of gastric acid. The customary time to take this medication is in the morning. If your physician

133

recommends taking the dose at another time of day or if your work schedule means that your first meal of the day is not breakfast, you should still take the preparation 30 to 60 minutes before a meal. If the medication is taken and not followed by a meal, it will have little effect.

Some patients may have to take this medication twice daily. If this is the case for you, then the first dose can be taken before breakfast and a second dose taken 30 to 60 minutes before the evening meal.

Notify Our Office If

● You have any questions about the timing of this medication.

Histamine-H$_2$ Acid-Blocking Drugs

Patient and Caregiver's Guide

General Information

Histamine-H$_2$ acid-blocking drugs are powerful agents for the suppression of gastric acid formation. They are used in the treatment of gastroesophageal reflux disease (GERD) and peptic ulcer, and they are part of the regimen for the eradication of *Helicobacter pylori*. They are less-powerful drugs than proton pump inhibitors, but they are effective for many people in relieving symptoms and healing their disease. They are also far less expensive than proton pump inhibitors.

Some are available as over-the-counter preparations and may be purchased without prescription. The preparations that are available include cimetidine (Tagamet), famotidine (Pepcid), nizatidine (Axid), and ranitidine (Zantac).

Peptic Ulcer Disease

Patient and Caregiver's Guide

General Information

An *ulcer* in the stomach or duodenum means that a hole has appeared in the lining of the stomach or small intestine near where it meets the stomach membrane. This hole extends deep enough into the wall of the organ so that healing produces a scar. Lesser degrees of inflammation of the lining, those that heal without the formation of a scar, are *gastritis* or *gastric erosions*. In younger patients, peptic ulcers are more commonly located in the duodenum, which is the first portion of the small intestine just beyond the stomach. In older patients, ulceration in the stomach itself becomes more common.

Typically ulcers present with burning pain that occurs in the front of the abdomen between the sternum (breast bone) and the navel. It is worse when the stomach is empty, and it is made better by eating or taking an antacid. Many patients do not have typical pain. A few may have no pain at all. Gastric (stomach) ulcers, which are most common in elderly patients, are a little less typical in their presentation. The pain may not be burning, the location is not so precise, and relief with food is less consistent.

Gastritis seems to render the lining of the stomach vulnerable to the development of ulcers. Gastritis can increase steadily in frequency with age as a result of an infection in the stomach. It is also particularly common in people taking aspirin-like anti-inflammatory drugs. This is a likely explanation for the increased occurrence of gastric ulcers in elderly patients.

Confirmation of the presence of an ulcer is important. This is particularly true, if it is a gastric ulcer. Cancers of the stomach can often mimic gastric ulcers, and they require different treatment. Although gastric ulcers may appear to be simple ulcers, a biopsy is usually performed to ensure that a tumor is not present. Often a biopsy is done to look for a type of infection that is often associated with peptic ulcers and gastritis. The treatment includes antibiotics, if this infection is present.

Important Points In Treatment

The treatment of ulceration in the stomach or duodenum involves the use of drugs. These may be drugs to suppress the production of acid, to neutralize acid, to treat infection in the stomach, or to protect the lining membrane from the effects of acid. The use of these drugs, either alone or in combination, has been highly effective, and surgery for ulcers, which used to be common, is now kept for the treatment of complications.

Once they occur, ulcers are likely to recur after healing. To prevent this, one takes lower doses of acid-suppressing drugs nightly after the ulcer heals. Treating the infection associated with peptic ulcers and gastritis is essential to prevent recurrence.

Complications

The complications of peptic ulcers are bleeding, perforation through the wall of the stomach or duodenum, scarring, and failure to respond to treatment. Because some people feel no pain or discomfort with an ulcer, they may have a complication as their first symptom.

Notify Our Office If

- You experience the onset of pain or burning in the stomach.
- You have any evidence of bleeding from the stomach. Blood in vomitus may be red but may also resemble coffee grounds. Blood in the stool often changes the feces so that they appear black and tarry.

Upper Gastrointestinal Tract Bleeding

Patient and Caregiver's Guide ■ ■ ■

General Information

Bleeding from the upper gastrointestinal tract is not a problem of aging, but it is a common problem in elderly patients. The bleeding may come from any site, from the nose to the upper portions of the small intestine. Most often the problem is from the stomach, caused by either ulcerations, ulcers in the stomach wall, or gastritis (inflammation of the wall of the stomach). Other possible sources are bleeding duodenal ulcers, bleeding esophageal varices (enlarged veins in the esophagus that occur in persons with cirrhosis), or arteriovenous malformations (abnormal connections between the arteries and the veins in the bowel wall that occur with aging). Much less frequently, cancer of the stomach or esophagus, nosebleeds, or bleeding from the lung is the cause.

If the bleeding is rapid, one may vomit bright red blood or blood that looks like coffee grounds as a result of exposure of the blood to acid in the stomach. Rapid bleeding may also stimulate rapid transport of the blood down the gastrointestinal tract so that it appears as red blood in the stool or as a black, tarry stool. During its stay in the digestive tract, blood turns black and sticky (tarry). If the bleeding is slow and the amounts are small, there may be no visible blood in the stool. Chemical testing is needed to detect its presence. This sort of blood is occult (hidden). Occasionally, the bleeding is so slow and intermittent that anemia is the only finding.

When upper gastrointestinal tract bleeding occurs quickly enough and in visible amounts, it is an urgent problem to report to your physician. Do not neglect even slow bleeding, even though it is not an emergency. The goal is to find the bleeding source and to stop the bleeding without the need for transfusion or surgery, if possible. Generally, the earlier that one can start treatment, the greater the likelihood that it will be successful.

Important Points In Treatment

Most bleeding from the gastrointestinal tract stops on its own. A search is undertaken by your physician for the cause of the bleeding to try to prevent future episodes. If the bleeding does not stop, techniques are available to the gastroenterologist or the radiologist to control the bleeding. If these are not successful, surgery may be needed, although resorting to surgery is uncommon.

Notify Our Office If

- You have any evidence of bleeding from the stomach. Blood in vomitus may be red but may also resemble coffee grounds. Blood in the stool often changes the feces so that they appear black and tarry.

Lower Gastrointestinal Tract Bleeding

Patient and Caregiver's Guide

General Information

Bleeding from the lower gastrointestinal tract is a problem of aging. The bleeding may come from any site in the large intestine, rectum, or anus. The blood may appear bright red, maroon, dark, or even black. Clots may or may not be visible. During its stay in the digestive tract, blood turns black and sticky. Physicians describe it as tarry, and that is an apt description. If the bleeding is slow and the amounts are small, there may be no visible blood in the stool. Chemical testing is needed to detect its presence. This sort of blood is occult (hidden). Occasionally, the bleeding is so slow and intermittent that anemia is the only finding.

It may be difficult to distinguish upper gastrointestinal tract bleeding, involving rapid passage of blood through the intestine, from lower tract bleeding. It may also be difficult to distinguish the source of bleeding if the bleeding is very slow and only occult blood or anemia is present.

Lower intestinal tract bleeding may be as simple as a bleeding hemorrhoid, or it may be a much more serious problem. Bleeding can occur from diverticula, which are small outpouchings in the wall of the large intestine; from arteriovenous malformations, which are abnormal connections between the arteries and the veins in the bowel wall that occur with aging; from colitis or other kinds of inflammation and infection; or from tumors, which may be either benign or malignant (cancer). In some people, no source can be found. Lower tract bleeding is serious and an urgent problem until proven otherwise. It is an error to ascribe a little blood to a hemorrhoid and neglect to investigate further.

Important Points In Treatment

Most bleeding from the gastrointestinal tract stops on its own. A search is undertaken by your physician for the cause of the

---

bleeding to try to prevent future episodes. If the bleeding does not stop, techniques are available to the gastroenterologist or the radiologist to control the bleeding. If these are not successful, surgery may be needed, although resorting to surgery is uncommon.

Notify Our Office If

- You have any evidence or suspicion of bleeding from the gastrointestinal tract. It is an error to ascribe a little blood seen in the stool or on toilet paper to a hemorrhoid and not investigate further.

Inflammatory Bowel Disease

Patient and Caregiver's Guide ▪ ▪ ▪

General Information

Colitis is an inflammation in the colon, and *ileitis* is an inflammation in the small intestine. *Inflammatory bowel disease* is the term used to describe the inflammatory diseases of the bowel, for which the cause is unknown.

Although inflammatory bowel disease regularly affects the young, there is also a late occurrence between ages 50 and 60. It is possible for elderly patients to have a first attack of inflammatory bowel disease. When the disease occurs for the first time in elderly patients, it often follows a more severe and progressive course.

Inflammatory bowel disease may remain confined to the colon (the large intestine) or to the small intestine, or it may affect both areas of the intestinal tract. Problems may occur outside the gastrointestinal tract. These extraintestinal problems may include the skin rashes, joint pain, eye pain, and liver problems.

Ulcerative colitis affects the colon and causes diarrhea and rectal bleeding. A change in bowel habit, particularly when associated with bleeding, should be reported to your physician promptly.

When the inflammation involves the small intestine or the small and large intestines combined, it is known as Crohn's disease.

Important Points In Treatment

Treatment involves the use of drugs to reduce the inflammation and to permit the colon and/or the small intestine to heal. Treatment often suppresses the disease, but it does not result in complete healing. Continued treatment is necessary to hold the symptoms at bay.

Complications

Complications, including severe toxic changes, perforation of the intestine, and scarring, can occur. Complications may require the intervention of the surgeon to resolve the difficulties.

Diet

It is wise to avoid milk and milk products, which are digested poorly in the diseased intestine.

Notify Our Office If

- You have a change in bowel habit, particularly when associated with bleeding.

143

Irritable Bowel Syndrome (IBS)

Patient and Caregiver's Guide ▪▪▪

General Information

The normal function of the digestive tract is marvelously coordinated. Food and fluids enter at the top for digestion and absorption. The waste moves smoothly down the digestive tract for timely elimination. Not surprisingly, in some people, a certain amount of incoordination in this process occurs. In many cases this is a result of an abnormality in visceral sensation. *Visceral sensation* is a term used to describe how the intestines' viscera perceive what is happening to them. These people do not have changes in their anatomy as a cause of this difficulty, nor do they have ulcers, tumors, or inflammation. This may involve the colon (the large intestine). The change is in function; hence, it is called *functional bowel disease*. Other names are *irritable colon syndrome, irritable bowel syndrome,* and *mucous colitis.*

Irritable colon syndrome can affect persons of any age. Elderly patients are not exempt. It is variable in its occurrence. Patients commonly experience long periods that are symptom free, punctuated by attacks of the problem that may last for days, weeks, or occasionally months. Although stress seems to initiate the attack, it is less likely that it is the cause; stress simply makes an underlying problem slightly worse so that it becomes apparent.

Irritable colon syndrome presents as a change in bowel habit, most often diarrhea, although diarrhea alternating with constipation does occur. Many people also experience a crampy abdominal pain, although a pain of this variety also occurs with simple diarrhea. Attacks are often abrupt in onset.

Important Points In Treatment

Treatment involves using medications to attempt to normalize the digestive tract function. If cramps are a problem, antispasmodic drugs are often helpful. If painless diarrhea is a problem, antidiarrheal drugs may correct the symptoms. The addition of a fiber supplement to the diet often benefits patients whose difficulty follows either pattern.

These are symptomatic treatments. When stress plays a role in the development and continuation of the problem, programs and medications for stress management are helpful.

Selection of the proper drug is essential because the treatment of painless diarrhea may worsen painful irritable colon syndrome, and the reverse is true as well. Your physician will discuss with you the potential diagnoses and needed tests.

There are drugs available that can normalize the sensory abnormality that underlies irritable bowel syndrome in many patients. Because the sensory abnormality is not the only cause of irritable bowel syndrome, these drugs are not effective in everyone. Treatment of this sort often involves the use of drugs also with central nervous system effects. These drugs are used in patients suffering from depression. It must be clear that depression and irritable bowel syndrome are not related.

Another drug, Zelnorm, may be useful in patients with constipation as the predominant symptom of their irritable bowel syndrome. Studies using this drug thus far have been limited to women. The drug is not helpful in patients with diarrhea and, in fact, may lead to a complication of dehydration in those patients.

 ## Notify Our Office If

- You have a change in bowel habit.

Functional Gastrointestinal Disease

Patient and Caregiver's Guide

General Information

The normal function of the digestive tract is marvelously coordinated. Food and fluids enter at the top for digestion and absorption. The waste moves smoothly down the digestive tract for timely elimination. Not surprisingly, in some people a certain amount of incoordination in this process occurs. These people do not have changes in their anatomy as a cause of this difficulty, and they have no ulcer, tumor, or inflammation. This may involve the esophagus (the swallowing tube), the stomach, the small intestine, the colon (the large intestine), or the gallbladder and biliary ducts. The change is in function; hence, it is called *functional gastrointestinal disease*. Other names include *noncardiac chest pain, functional dyspepsia, biliary dyskinesia, irritable colon syndrome, irritable bowel syndrome, mucous colitis,* and *proctalgia fugax.*

Functional gastrointestinal disease can affect persons of any age. Elderly patients are not exempt. It is variable in its occurrence. Patients commonly experience long periods that are symptom free, punctuated by attacks of the problem that may last for days, weeks, or, occasionally, months. Although stress seems to initiate the attack, it is less likely that it is the cause; stress simply makes an underlying problem slightly worse so that it becomes apparent.

Noncardiac chest pain resembles the discomfort that occurs with angina or a heart attack, but noncardiac chest pain comes from the esophagus. It is a common problem. Diagnosis requires special testing of the function of the esophagus.

Functional dyspepsia resembles the discomfort associated with gastritis (inflammation in the stomach) or peptic ulcers. It occurs in the absence of ulcers or inflammation. It is often called *nonulcer dyspepsia.*

Biliary dyskinesia is a problem that resembles the difficulty that occurs with gallstones. There is pain and discomfort in the

Constipation

Patient and Caregiver's Guide ■ ■ ■

General Information

Constipation is the slowing of bowel function. Bowel movements become less frequent. With constipation, people also strain at the time of the bowel movement, pass hard dry stools, and have the sensation of an incomplete bowel movement. Some people also experience an urge to have a bowel movement but are unable to carry it through. Many people will have only one or two of these symptoms.

By itself, constipation is responsible for only a few problems. It may cause the development of fecal impaction and straining of stool. The hard stools sometimes associated with constipation may give rise to fissure or cause hemorrhoids to bleed. The straining associated with constipation may be a cause of the prolapse of hemorrhoids.

Constipation receives the blame for many other systemic symptoms. Most of these are nonspecific, such as fatigue, insomnia, fullness, and loss of appetite. It is not likely that the constipation is a direct cause of this sort of symptom.

For most people, bowel function and its frequency are regular in occurrence and timing during the day. The range of normal frequency is wide, from three bowel movements daily to three times a week; both greater and lesser frequency rates occur in normal people.

Far more significant is a change in the *customary* frequency, regularity, or both. However, such a change is only a clue, not a diagnosis. There are many innocent causes for a change in bowel habit. These include changes in diet, both in composition and amount, including the addition or substitution of milk, fiber, fresh fruit, and the like. Abrupt changes in exercise, such as those caused by illness, can also change function. Even gravity seems important, and prolonged bed rest alone can slow bowel function. Less frequent, but much more serious, are changes in bowel habit caused by thyroid disease or complications from diabetes, heart failure, or other problems. Differentiation of simple constipation from more complicated medical problems is the physician's task.

Although relief of symptoms greatly improves comfort, your physician is equally concerned with the cause of the constipation. Tumors and narrowing of the colon may also give rise to constipation-like symptoms. Do not assume that constipation is harmless.

Important Points In Treatment

The best treatment for constipation is treatment of the underlying cause. Laxatives, however effective, remain the second-best treatment. Controlling symptoms is never as effective as curing their cause. Many different classes of cathartics are available without the need for a prescription. These include potent agents that can stimulate bowel action in most individuals, despite the mechanism of their constipation. Such therapy provides only temporary relief of symptoms. Selection of a laxative that has a mechanism of action that helps return the bowel habit to normal is a far more appropriate treatment. Your physician remains your best guide to this selection.

Notify Our Office If

- You experience a change in bowel habit. The best treatment for constipation is treatment of the underlying cause.

Fecal Impaction

Patient and Caregiver's Guide ■ ■ ■

General Information

It is possible for enough slowing to occur in the movements of the intestine that the contents become excessively dried and hard. If this occurs at the outlet, just above the anus, fecal impaction may develop. Impaction is a mass of fecal material that is too large or too firm, or both, to pass through the anus.

Impaction may form in a setting of simple constipation. It is also common in association with neurologic problems that extend to involve the nerves and muscles in the pelvis. Strokes and dementia are common antecedents. Because many of these problems occur with aging, the problem of fecal impaction is frequent in elderly patients.

Symptoms associated with fecal impaction are highly variable. Some patients feel a sense of fullness, others of urgency, and others of an incomplete bowel movement when they finish evacuating. Some patients may have no sensation that there is anything wrong at all.

Patients with impaction may complain of constipation. Although it seems paradoxical, some patients with impaction complain of diarrhea. Watery or soft feces pass around the impaction, seeming to be diarrhea. The impaction may so alter the dynamics in the rectum that patients have incontinence.

Important Points In Treatment

Your physician will find impaction at the time of physical examination when placing a gloved finger in the rectum. Treatment of impaction is to break it up or soften it with oil enemas to permit passage of the feces. Often your physician may prescribe a thorough cleansing of the colon, using an oral solution that washes through the colon or a series of enemas. After this, it may require regular treatment with medications to soften the stools.

It is far better to prevent the formation of impaction than to have to treat it. Maintain exercise to speed the passage of feces

157

through the intestine. Avoid long periods of relative dehydration. Take adequate fluids throughout the day. Stool softeners may be used, and the addition of supplemental fiber to the diet helps ensure the rapid transit of feces and keeps it from drying out excessively.

Laxatives, suppositories, and enemas should be used with caution and preferably at the direction of a physician.

Notify Our Office If

- You experience a change in bowel habit. The best treatment for impaction is treatment of the underlying cause.

Diarrhea

Patient and Caregiver's Guide

General Information

When bowel movements become unusually frequent, loose and watery, or both, it is diarrhea. The range of normal for bowel habit is highly variable among individuals. Generally, if an individual is having more than three bowel movements daily, particularly if they are loose and if the volume seems large, there is cause to investigate the possibility of diarrhea. If a patient has a change in customary bowel habit, although it may not exceed these limits, there is cause for further investigation.

Diarrhea is not a phenomenon of aging, but it is a frequent problem in elderly patients. Diarrhea can cause dehydration because of excessive loss of fluids and salts, and this is less well tolerated by elderly patients. Prompt diagnosis and treatment can avoid these possible complications.

It is difficult to know when it is necessary to call on a physician for help with a problem that is so common and so often self-limited. As a rule, seek help if diarrhea occurs in association with fever, chills, or a skin rash or if blood is present in the stool. Patients who are diabetic or who are taking heart medications may experience complications earlier and with less diarrhea than people who are otherwise healthy. They are a high-risk group.

Important Points In Treatment

Mild diarrhea is most often a self-limited disease and resolves on its own. The use of fluids with some salt in them for supplements may make you more comfortable. Cola drinks seem particularly useful in this regard. They contain a small amount of potassium, which is a salt lost with the diarrhea. They are palatable and well tolerated, even if you have had difficulty with nausea and vomiting. Special oral salt replacement solutions are available, but these are rarely necessary in adults.

If you are in a high-risk category or if the diarrhea is unusually severe and persistent, hospitalization may be necessary to permit intravenous fluid administration.

Notify Our Office If

- You have diarrhea in association with fever, chills, or a skin rash, or if there is blood in the stool.
- You have symptoms of diarrhea and are diabetic or on heart medications. Patients who are diabetic or who are taking heart medications may experience complications earlier and with less diarrhea than people who are otherwise healthy. They are a high-risk group.
- You have chronic diarrhea. This is diarrhea that has been present for more than 5 days or is a recurrent event, even if there are intervals of normal bowel habit.

Enemas

Patient and Caregiver's Guide ■ ■ ■

General Information

Any injection of fluid into the rectum is an enema. It can be used for the administration of drugs, for the purpose of diagnosis, in preparation for diagnostic procedures, or, most commonly, for the stimulation of a bowel movement.

Properly done, an enema is not harmful to one's health or the colon (the large intestine). Improperly done or done with toxic or harsh constituents, it can harm the intestine, one's general health, or both. In certain diseases of the rectum and large intestine, enemas are potentially harmful.

Enemas intended for therapy for diseases should be used only as prescribed by your physician. Many drugs that enter through the lower intestinal tract require careful regulation of dosage. Diagnostic enemas are always used at the discretion of a physician.

Cleansing enemas have been a feature of personal hygiene for centuries. In the middle 1800s and early 1900s, there was a belief that toxic fermentations from the bacteria in the lower intestinal tract were responsible for many different illnesses and for ill health, in general. Thus, many people used frequent, even daily, cleansing enemas. There is no evidence that cleansing enemas are necessary or desirable for maintenance of good health and well-being. Generally, such cleansing is not harmful; it is just not necessary. Individuals who have become comfortable with the procedure may safely continue. Initiation of regular cleansing enemas is often not necessary.

Occasionally, enemas can be used to relieve simple constipation. Constipation that recurs and represents a change in bowel habit is a symptom that should be reported to your physician. Effective relief with an enema can mask a serious underlying health problem.

Important Points In Treatment

If you want to or you must use an enema, several points are important. Devices for administration should be cleaned to

161

the point of being sterile. It is possible to introduce infection with improperly cleaned administration devices. Many small-volume enemas and disposable administration kits are available at drugstores.

The volume of an enema should be carefully controlled. Rarely is more than 1 pint of enema fluid required, and 1 quart should be the absolute limit.

The fluid constituents should be mild and nontoxic. Tap-water enemas made with potable water involve few complications. Injury of the lining of the lower intestine has occurred from such innocent substances as soapsuds. Salt-containing enemas may be harmful in patients with heart disease. If you have any questions about the safety of using an enema, seek the advice of your physician. If you have a rectal abscess, fissure, or serious hemorrhoidal disease, an enema may cause pain or more serious consequences. Enemas may also be contraindicated in certain primary intestinal diseases.

 ## Notify Our Office If

- You have constipation that recurs. This represents a change in bowel habit.

Laxatives

Patient and Caregiver's Guide ▪ ▪ ▪

General Information

Normal bowel function is a concern that has captured human attention from time immemorial. Although at one time or another, many signs and symptoms associated with diseases were ascribed to simple constipation, constipation causes relatively few problems.

For most people, bowel function and its frequency are regular in occurrence and timing during the day. The range of normal frequency is wide, from three bowel movements daily to three times per week; both greater and lesser frequency rates occur in normal people.

Far more significant is a change in your customary frequency, regularity, or both. However, such a change is only a clue, not a diagnosis. There are many innocent causes for a change in bowel habit. These include changes in diet, both composition and amount, including the addition or substitution of milk, fiber, fresh fruit, and the like. Abrupt changes in exercise, such as those caused by illness, also can change function. Even gravity seems important, and prolonged bed rest alone can slow bowel function. Less frequent, but much more serious, are changes in bowel habit caused by thyroid disease or complications from diabetes, heart failure, or other problems. Differentiation of simple constipation from more complicated medical problems is the physician's task.

Important Points In Treatment

Treatment of simple constipation is most effective if it addresses the probable cause of the constipation. Laxative preparations are available in many varieties, including bulk-forming agents, saline (salt) lavages, chemical stimulants, contact stimulants (agents that have a direct effect when they contact the lining of the intestine), stool softeners, and saline cathartics (the traditional "dose of salts"). All can be effective in stimulating a bowel movement, but only the careful matching of a laxative with the cause of the constipation can provide a return to your normal bowel habit, after which the use of the laxative should be stopped altogether.

Prolonged use of a laxative, which is often the outcome of the selection of an improper one, may lead to unwanted side effects and complications. In effect, this is a form of laxative abuse. These complications can include weakness because of a loss of fluids and salts and the development of pigmentation in the lining of the large intestine, the colon.

Powerful cathartics of all classes are regularly available without prescription. Nonetheless, their appropriate use requires the same insight and understanding that are necessary to select from the many prescription-only drugs available for other diseases. Thus, your physician remains your most authoritative guide. Whenever possible, it is best to treat the underlying cause of the constipation and, if necessary, to select the laxative that reinforces the return to normal bowel habit.

Notify Our Office If

- You have any change in bowel habit. Far more significant is a change in your customary frequency or regularity, or both. Such a change is only a clue, not a diagnosis.

Fiber Therapy

Patient and Caregiver's Guide

General Information

Dietary fiber is a plant product that is commonly present in food but cannot be digested by the intestinal tract. It adds bulk to the diet but does not offer nutrition. Much time and money are spent by the food industry to eliminate fiber from prepared foods. Fiber is important in the normal function of the intestinal tract.

It is easier for food and other nutrients to move down the intestinal tract if there is also sufficient bulk. The effect is much like what we all experience with a toothpaste tube. When the tube is new and full of toothpaste, it takes little effort to squeeze it out. When the tube is nearly empty, it needs to be rolled up and pressed hard to get even a little toothpaste out. When your intestine is full, it takes little effort to move the contents on. When it is relatively empty, the intestine must struggle and squeeze to move its contents.

This increase in squeeze that is needed to move material in a nearly empty intestine may cause the formation of diverticula, cramps, and other symptoms. Changes in the intestine from this can take a long time to develop. These changes may not be reversible.

Important Points In Treatment

Fiber therapy is directed toward replacement of fiber that food processing has removed from our diet. This may be accomplished by eating foods naturally high in fiber content or by taking a fiber supplement daily.

The benefit of natural supplementation of fiber by eating foods with high fiber content is that it avoids the cost of medication. The problem is that there are relatively few foods high enough in fiber content, and a steady diet of these foods becomes monotonous. Fiber is derived from plants. The cereal plants are particularly high in fiber. Whole wheat, wheat bran, and oats are excellent sources. Most other vegetables contain some fiber, but it is difficult to regularly eat enough vegetables to maintain an adequate fiber supplement. Except for the daily use of high-fiber cereals for breakfast, dietary supplementation of fiber tends to be inconsistent.

A number of fiber supplements are designed to be taken as medicine rather than food. These include natural compounds, usually the husk of the psyllium seed, and synthetic compounds, including polycarbophil and methylcellulose. These compounds work well but must be taken with adequate fluids to prevent them from clumping into a plug in the intestine. Many are designed to be mixed with water or other drinks and are flavored. Some of these preparations are available in capsule or caplet form. These must be taken with adequate fluids, usually at least 12 ounces for them to be fully effective to prevent complications. These compounds must be taken regularly to be effective.

Notify Our Office If

- You have difficulty with constipation.
- You experience rectal bleeding.
- You have cramping abdominal discomfort.

Hepatitis A

Patient and Caregiver's Guide

General Information

Hepatitis A is a virus that can cause injury to the liver. This injury can appear as jaundice (yellow eyes and skin) and abnormal liver blood tests. It can often occur in outbreaks of several persons.

Hepatitis A is spread by the fecal-oral route, meaning a person can spread it if they have a bowel movement and do not wash their hands correctly. Commonly, outbreaks are centered at either a restaurant where an employee is infected or at family gatherings where contaminated food is served.

Important Points In Treatment

Hepatitis A is usually nonfatal. There are no medications to treat the virus because the vast majority of affected persons get over the illness on their own.

Very rarely hepatitis A infection can lead to liver failure requiring a liver transplant. This is uncommon, and most therapy is directed at making a patient feel better while they are getting over the disease. Hepatitis A does not cause chronic liver disease or cirrhosis. There is a vaccine for hepatitis A, which is recommended for persons traveling to areas overseas where hepatitis A is common, persons exposed to sewage as part of their job, and persons with chronic liver disease.

Call Our Office If

- Your skin or eyes have become yellow (jaundice).
- You think you were exposed to a hepatitis A outbreak.
- You will be traveling to an area overseas where hepatitis A is common.

Hepatitis B

Patient and Caregiver's Guide

General Information

Hepatitis B is a virus that causes injury to the liver. It can cause both acute injury (viral hepatitis) and chronic injury (cirrhosis).

Hepatitis B is a virus that can be spread by contact with blood from another person who has hepatitis B or by contact with body fluids from a person who is infected. In the past (prior to the 1970s), it was most often acquired by a blood transfusion. Today, acquiring it through a transfusion is rare.

Acute hepatitis B often presents with jaundice (yellow eyes and skin), nausea, fatigue, and loss of interest in smoking (in patients who smoke). Chronic hepatitis B usually causes no symptoms, unless a patient develops cirrhosis. Occasionally, it can cause a rash and kidney problems.

There are medications that can treat hepatitis B, including Interferon (an injection) and lamivudine, adefovir, and tenofovir (pills), with more medications to be introduced in the future. Treatment is long term, from 6 months to 2 or more years. Not every person who has chronic hepatitis B needs treatment; however, some of the medications cannot be used in some patients because of side effects.

There is a vaccine for hepatitis B, and all children today receive this vaccine. It is recommended for health care workers, travelers to areas where hepatitis B is common, persons living with someone who has chronic hepatitis B, and persons with chronic liver disease.

Important Points In Treatment

Therapy for hepatitis B is a long-term proposition. Interferon is generally used for 12 weeks or more, and lamivudine or adefovir are used for upwards of 2 years or more. It is important to not miss doses of your medication.

Notify Our Office If

- Your skin or eyes have become yellow (jaundice).
- You think you were exposed to hepatitis B.
- You will be traveling overseas to an area where hepatitis B is common.

Hepatitis C

Patient and Caregiver's Guide

General Information

Hepatitis C is a virus that causes injury to the liver. It can cause both acute injury (viral hepatitis) and chronic injury (cirrhosis).

Hepatitis C is a virus that can be spread by contact with blood from another person who has hepatitis C or by contact with body fluids from a person who is infected. In the past (prior to the 1970s), it was most often acquired by a blood transfusion. Today, acquiring through transfusion is rare.

Acute hepatitis C is rarely seen because patients often do not become jaundiced (yellow skin or eyes). Most patients who have chronic hepatitis C may not remember when they contracted it years prior. Chronic hepatitis C usually causes no symptoms, unless a patient develops cirrhosis. Occasionally, it can cause a rash and kidney problems.

There are medications that can treat hepatitis C, namely interferon (PEG-Intron or Pegasys) and ribavirin (Rebetol or Copegus). Interferon is an injection taken once a week, whereas ribavirin is a pill taken daily. Not every person who has chronic hepatitis C needs treatment; however, some of the medications cannot be used in some patients because of side effects.

There is not yet a vaccine for hepatitis C. It is recommended that anyone with chronic hepatitis C be vaccinated against hepatitis A and B, if he or she is not already immune to them.

Important Points In Treatment

Therapy for hepatitis C is a long-term proposition. Interferon and ribavirin are used for between 6 months and 1 year. It is important to try to take each dose of your medication.

Notify Our Office If

- Your skin or eyes have become yellow (jaundice).
- You think you were exposed to hepatitis C.

Cirrhosis of the Liver

Patient and Caregiver's Guide

General Information

Cirrhosis of the liver is severe scarring of the liver that can lead to loss of liver function, bleeding problems, difficulty with memory and thinking (encephalopathy), and retaining fluid (ascites or edema). It can be caused by many liver diseases.

Cirrhosis is also referred to as "end-stage liver disease" and can be caused by many diseases, including alcohol overuse, viral hepatitis (hepatitis B or C), medications, immune problems (autoimmune hepatitis, primary sclerosing cholangitis, primary biliary cirrhosis), and too much iron (hereditary hemochromatosis), among others. Many of these problems do not cause symptoms until a person develops cirrhosis.

The symptoms of cirrhosis can vary from one person to another and can include the following:
- Retaining fluid in the abdomen (ascites)
- Retaining fluid in the legs (edema)
- Difficulty thinking or with memory (encephalopathy)
- Very easy bruising
- Muscle loss
- Enlarged veins in the esophagus (varices)
- Cancer of the liver.

Cirrhosis is not thought to be reversible, even if the underlying condition is cured. Its progression can be slowed down, however, if the underlying condition is cured or brought under control. The only cure for cirrhosis is a liver transplant.

Important Points In Treatment

Therapy for cirrhosis revolves around treating symptoms and preventing problems. Fluid in the abdomen or legs can be treated with water pills (diuretics) and by decreasing salt in the diet. Difficulty with thinking can be treated with medications called Lactulose and neomycin and sometimes by restricting protein in the diet. Enlarged veins in the esophagus do not cause symptoms

171

but can bleed suddenly. A person would vomit blood or pass blood from the rectum if this happens. Your doctor can look for these veins by looking in the esophagus with an endoscope and he or she can treat them by placing rubber bands on them or by using a medication called a beta-blocker.

Notify Our Office If

- You suddenly develop swelling in the legs or your abdomen seems to be becoming larger.
- You suddenly develop difficulty thinking or with memory (a patient may not realize this, but caregivers will notice it).
- You begin vomiting blood or passing blood from the rectum.

Esophago-Gastro-Duodenoscopy (EGD)

Patient and Caregiver's Guide

General Information

Esophago-gastro-duodenoscopy, commonly called EGD, is a procedure that permits the physician to inspect the esophagus (the swallowing tube), the stomach, and the first portion of the small intestine called the duodenum. It is an outpatient procedure that can be done in an endoscopy center, an ambulatory surgical center, a physician's office, or at a hospital. In some circumstances it may be directly scheduled by your physician, although there are times when a visit to the endoscopist is required some days before the procedure is performed.

This procedure is commonly performed on patients with gastroesophageal reflux disease, difficulty swallowing, unexplained chest pain, upper gastrointestinal bleeding, and ulcer-like pain. There are many other reasons why this procedure may be recommended.

The preparation for the procedure is simple. Usually, patients are asked to have nothing to eat after midnight prior to the procedure. This ensures that the stomach will be empty and that the physician can get a good view that is unobscured by food. Prior to the procedure, the physician will explain it, including its possible complications, and he or she will request that a consent form be signed to perform the procedure. Although this is not a surgical procedure, it is an invasive procedure, so an operative consent is obtained.

Prior to the procedure, an intravenous infusion is started. Patients usually receive a gargle or a spray of a topical anesthetic to numb the throat and reduce the problem of the gag reflex. Be sure to inform your physician of any allergic reactions to any anesthetic drugs. To assist with the performance of the procedure, patients are often offered conscious sedation with intravenous medications. This is a mild form of anesthesia that does not put the patient to sleep but relaxes them and makes the procedure

173

more comfortable. Often conscious sedation will produce amnesia for the procedure in many patients who may not remember that the procedure has been performed. Additional medication may be administered during the procedure.

During the procedure the physician will be able to look at the inside of the esophagus, the stomach, and the duodenum. Air may be injected to permit the view of all of the areas of the stomach. It is also possible to wash off areas of the stomach through the endoscope. It is possible to remove small samples of tissue (obtain a biopsy) through the endoscope. This is painless. It is possible to do injections through the endoscope. This may be done to control bleeding. Bleeding may also be controlled with devices passed through the endoscope, which can cauterize the bleeding vessel with heat, electricity, or light. There are times when a device may be added to the endoscope to permit a rubber band to be placed around a bleeding vessel to control the hemorrhage.

Following the procedure, patients are usually monitored in a recovery room for about 1 hour. This permits the conscious sedation to wear off. Once the patient is fully recovered he or she will be discharged to go home. Because of the conscious sedation, the patient will not be able to drive an automobile for the remainder of the day. The lingering effect of the conscious sedation may affect judgment, and patients are warned to not undertake business activities for the remainder of the day. The effects of these drugs have usually completely dissipated by the following day.

The physician will usually ask whether you will permit a person accompanying you to be informed about the findings obtained during the procedure. This is because the lingering effect of the conscious sedation may impair your ability to remember what has been found. You will usually be asked to return to your physician following the procedure. The return visit will be delayed at least several days to permit reports about any tissue removed at the time of the procedure to be obtained.

Endoscopic Retrograde Cholangiopancreatography (ERCP)

Patient and Caregiver's Guide

General Information

Endoscopic retrograde cholangiopancreatography (ERCP) is a procedure performed with an endoscope passed through the mouth, the esophagus (the swallowing tube), the stomach, and into the small intestine. The physician will attempt to locate the opening of the common bile duct, where it enters the duodenum. The physician may then pass a small tube into the duct for diagnostic studies or treatment.

It is possible to inject dye through this tube to outline the bile duct and the pancreatic duct on an x-ray and to look for the presence of gallstones or some other obstruction. It is also possible to pass other devices through the endoscope into the ducts to permit the opening of the duct into the small intestine to be enlarged, a sphincterotomy, or to permit the extraction of a gallstone trapped in the duct. It is also possible to identify and sometimes to sample mass lesions where the possibility of a tumor is suspected.

ERCP may be performed as an outpatient procedure; however, it frequently requires at least a short stay in the hospital. It is performed at a facility equipped with an x-ray and thus is not performed at a physician's office.

Preparation for ERCP involves abstaining from food and drink from midnight the night before the procedure. This permits the endoscope to be inserted into a stomach that is free of food. Prior to the procedure the physician will explain the procedure, why it is being done, and what the possible complications are. This is an invasive procedure and will require the patient's informed consent. There are a number of serious complications that can occur as a result of the procedure, and these will be discussed fully.

Prior to the procedure, an intravenous infusion is started. Patients usually receive a gargle or a spray of a topical anesthetic

175

to get in the throat and reduce the problem of the gag reflex. The physician should be informed of allergies to any anesthetic drugs. To assist with the performance of the procedure patients are often offered conscious sedation. This is a mild form of anesthesia that does not put the patient to sleep but relaxes them and makes the procedure more comfortable. Often conscious sedation will produce amnesia for the procedure in many patients who do not remember that the procedure has been performed. In some circumstances when the procedure is expected to be prolonged, anesthesia provided by an anesthesiologist may be recommended.

Following the procedure, patients are usually monitored in a recovery room. This permits the conscious sedation or the anesthesia to wear off. Once the patient is fully recovered, he or she may be discharged to go home. Overnight stays in the hospital are not uncommon. If complications occur, a more prolonged stay is possible. Because of the conscious sedation, the patient will not be able to drive an automobile for the remainder of the day. The lingering effect of the conscious sedation may affect judgment, and patients are warned to not undertake business activities for the remainder of the day. The effects of these drugs have usually completely dissipated by the following day.

The physician will usually ask whether you will permit a person accompanying you to be informed about the findings obtained during the procedure. This is because the lingering effect of the conscious sedation may impair your ability to remember what has been found. You will usually be asked to return to your physician following the procedure. The return visit will be delayed at least several days to permit reports about any tissue removed at the time of the procedure to be obtained.

Colonoscopy

Patient and Caregiver's Guide

General Information

Colonoscopy is a procedure that permits the physician to examine the inside of the colon, the lower digestive tract. It may be performed to look for a source of abdominal pain, bleeding, or diarrhea, or to evaluate an abnormality that has been identified by one of the x-ray examinations. It is also performed in older patients as a screening test for colon polyps (benign tumors) or colon cancers.

It is an outpatient procedure that can be done in an endoscopy center, an ambulatory surgical center, a physician's office, or at a hospital. In some circumstances it may be directly scheduled by your physician, although there are times when a visit to the endoscopist is required some days before the procedure is performed.

Preparation for the procedure involves cleansing the colon to facilitate its examination. A number of different approaches are used to cleanse the colon. The physician performing the endoscopy will see that you are instructed about the preparation procedure that he or she uses. The preparation often involves a liquid diet for a day or more before the procedure. Patients should avoid eating or drinking foods that contain red dyes or red-colored materials. This would prevent any residual from being mistaken for blood when the colon examination is performed. In addition, patients are asked to refrain from eating or drinking after midnight the night before the procedure is scheduled.

Prior to the procedure an intravenous infusion is started. Be sure to inform your physician, if you are allergic to any anesthetic drugs. To assist with the performance of the procedure, patients are often offered conscious sedation. This is a mild form of anesthesia that does not put the patient to sleep but relaxes them and makes the procedure more comfortable. Often conscious sedation will produce amnesia for the procedure. In some circumstances when the procedure is expected to be prolonged, anesthesia provided by an anesthesiologist may be recommended.

During the procedure the physician will be able to look at the inside of the colon. Air may be injected to permit the viewing of all of the areas of the colon. It is also possible to wash off areas of the colon through the endoscope. It is possible to remove small samples of tissue (obtain a biopsy) through the endoscope. This is painless. It is possible to do injections through the endoscope. This may be done to control bleeding. Bleeding may also be controlled with devices passed through the endoscope, which can cauterize the bleeding vessel with heat, electricity, or light. If polyps (colon tumors) are seen, it may be possible to remove them with the biopsy forceps or with a wire snare. This is painless. These tumors will then be retrieved so that they may be examined by the pathologist.

To complete the examination of the entire colon the physician will need to manipulate the instrument to move around the corners. To facilitate this the patient may be asked to change position, or the endoscopy assistant may apply pressure to your abdomen.

Following the procedure patients are usually monitored in a recovery room for about 1 hour. This permits the conscious sedation to wear off. Once the patient is fully recovered, he or she will be discharged to go home. Because of the conscious sedation, the patient will not be able to drive an automobile for the remainder of the day. The lingering effect of the conscious sedation may affect judgment, and patients are warned to not undertake business activities for the remainder of the day. The effects of these drugs have usually completely dissipated by the following day.

The physician will usually ask whether you will permit a person accompanying you to be informed about the findings obtained during the procedure. This is because the lingering effect of the conscious sedation may impair your ability to remember what has been found. You will usually be asked to return to your physician following the procedure. The return visit will be delayed at least several days to permit reports about any tissue that is removed.

Flexible Sigmoidoscopy

Patient and Caregiver's Guide

General Information

Flexible sigmoidoscopy is a procedure that permits the physician to examine the rectum and the lower portion of the colon (the large intestine). It is commonly used to evaluate patients who have diarrhea, anemia, rectal bleeding, or abdominal pain. It may also be used as a screening test in older individuals to look for the possible development of colon polyps or colon cancer.

Flexible sigmoidoscopy is an outpatient procedure that may be performed at the physician's office, an endoscopy center, an ambulatory surgical center, or at the hospital. It does not require anesthesia or conscious sedation. In preparation for the procedure patients are asked to refrain from eating or drinking after midnight the evening before the procedure. A colon cleansing preparation is used. This commonly consists of several cleansing enemas and may involve the use of a cathartic as well. Your physician will see that you are instructed about the preparation that he or she customarily uses.

Because this is an invasive procedure, you will be asked to sign an informed consent form. Before signing this consent, the nature of the procedure, the reasons for doing the procedure, and the possible complications will be explained to you.

During the procedure the physician may inject air through the endoscope to help visualize the various areas of the colon and rectum. It is possible for the physician to wash off areas through the endoscope, and it is also possible to obtain samples of tissue through the endoscope. In addition, it is possible to remove polyps using biopsy forceps or a snare, usually with electrical cautery. In the event that bleeding is seen, it may be possible to stop the bleeding either with the application of heat, electro-cautery, or the use of light. It is also possible to inject through the endoscope and stop bleeding.

Following the procedure, as soon as you are stable you will be discharged to go home. An appointment is usually made for a follow-up visit when tissue has been removed for examination by a pathologist. It can take days for this examination to be completed.

CHAPTER 9

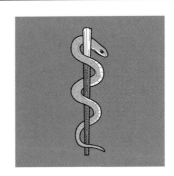
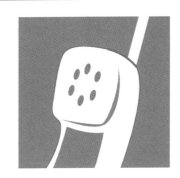

Cardiovascular Problems

Angina Pectoris

Patient and Caregiver's Guide

General Information

Coronary artery disease occurs with the development of hardening of the arteries that feed blood to the heart muscle. The deposits of cholesterol that harden these arteries also narrow the artery and limit the amount of blood that can flow through it. Exercise increases the heart rate. Normally, this results in an increase in blood flow through the coronary arteries to provide oxygen for the exercising heart's muscle. When this increase in blood flow fails to occur because of the narrowed arteries, pain in the chest—heart pain—is one result. This pain is called *angina pectoris*. The occurrence of artery narrowing rises with age. Coronary artery disease is a phenomenon of aging.

Typical anginal pain comes on with exercise and abates with rest. Emotional upset or a large meal, if it causes the heart rate to increase, counts as exercise. The pain is most often felt in the left side of the chest, in the front. It can spread to or occur in the neck, jaw, shoulder (usually left shoulder), and left arm. Cold weather seems to be associated with increased frequency and attacks of anginal pain.

Generally, patients with angina learn how much exercise they can tolerate without the development of painful discomfort in the chest. Angina can mimic pain caused by musculoskeletal abnormalities, arthritis, or muscle and joint strain in the muscles and bones, particularly of the chest. Conversely, pain from these sources can mimic angina. Angina-mimicking pain can also be a result of heartburn or esophageal inflammation or gallstone attacks and, on rare occasions, peptic ulcer discomfort. Because anginal pain implies a risk of sudden death, it is wise to have your physician evaluate new or recurrent chest pain.

Chest pain is not an inevitable accompaniment of a decrease in blood flow to the heart muscle. This is particularly true in the elderly, in whom heart attacks in the absence of chest pain are common. In these patients, shortness of breath or heart failure may be the presenting problem.

Important Points In Treatment

If angina pectoris is the diagnosis, a decision concerning its control depends on the extent of involvement of the coronary arteries in the narrowing process. Many patients receive treatment with medicines alone. Drugs called *vasodilators* help the arteries remain open as widely as possible. Nitroglycerin and its derivatives are most often used to dilate the coronary arteries, but a wide selection of other drug preparations (calcium channel blockers) is available for this purpose as well. In addition, drugs, usually beta blockers, are given to regulate the heartbeat. Low doses of aspirin may be given to act as a blood thinner and prevent the possible progression of the angina to a heart attack.

Much can be done to prevent anginal pain. Exercise and activity, which are important to maintain physical condition, should continue but should be kept to a level below that which triggers the anginal pain. Many tasks can be done without precipitating anginal attacks, if approached in a measured and thoughtful manner. Your physician can counsel you about the appropriateness of some forms of work or exercise.

Patients with angina have good and bad days. Exploit the good days and respect the bad ones. Be cautious when the weather adds to stress levels.

Notify Our Office If

- You experience pain in the chest. *New* pain or *recurring* pain is a real risk and a warning for urgent evaluation.
- You experience a change in pain in the chest. Pain that *changes* and *becomes unstable* often precedes a heart attack. Unstable pain may come on with less than the usual amount of exercise or sometimes without any exercise at all, while you are at rest or in bed. Its relief is less predictable, and it may persist for a longer interval.

Nitroglycerin Tablets

Patient and Caregiver's Guide

General Information

Nitroglycerin has long been used in the treatment of heart pain. It causes the arterial blood vessels to widen (dilate), thereby increasing the blood flow through them to the organ that they supply. This permits increased blood flow to the heart muscle, which, in turn, eases the pain from the heart.

Because heart pain tends to come on suddenly and without warning, treatment for it may require rapid administration of a drug to stop the pain. The most common form of nitroglycerin is the sublingual (under the tongue) form. Nitroglycerin tablets designed for this method of administration dissolve quickly and are absorbed into the blood circulation through the mucosa that forms the covering of the tongue and the lining of the mouth.

Many other forms of nitroglycerin are available. Some sprays may be applied under the tongue, which also provides rapid absorption. When patients have frequent or prolonged heart pain, the doctor may prescribe a long-acting oral preparation. Nitroglycerin is also made in a form that is absorbed slowly through the skin. Sometimes a paste is used for this purpose. This paste or ointment is applied directly to the skin. Another form is a patch that can be stuck directly onto the skin.

Each form of nitroglycerin has specific indications for its use. Your physician will discuss with you which form may be the most helpful for the kind of heart pain that you are experiencing.

Important Points in Therapy

Nitroglycerin, designed to be taken under the tongue, should be fresh. This medication can lose some of its potency with the passage of time. These tablets should be stored in the refrigerator with only a small quantity retained on the person. The tablets should be kept in their opaque container or dark brown bottle because they are light-sensitive. Unless you use a great deal

185

of the medicine in a short time, it is wise to ask for a limited prescription with some renewals so you can obtain fresh drug at regular intervals. The drug should be obtained about every 3 or 4 months to ensure its potency. The drug needs to be stored in a tightly closed vial.

Before taking the pill, the mouth should be moist. If it is dry, take a sip of water or other beverage and swallow the liquid. Then place the tablet under your tongue. Let the tablet sit there with your mouth closed until it has dissolved. Do not try to swallow the tablet. Do not drink, smoke, or chew until it is gone. Wait several minutes before taking a drink of water or other beverage.

A potent nitroglycerin tablet should give the feeling of a throbbing pulse and, in some patients, may cause a headache. One should also feel a slight tingling under the tongue as the tablet dissolves. This is a sign that the drug is active.

Notify Our Office If

- You experience chest pain.
- You do not experience a thumping pulse, a headache, or a tingling sensation when you use your sublingual (under the tongue) nitroglycerin tablets.

Nitroglycerin Spray

Patient and Caregiver's Guide ▪ ▪ ▪

General Information

Nitroglycerin has long been used in the treatment of heart pain. It causes the arterial blood vessels to widen (dilate), thereby increasing the blood flow through them to the organ that they supply. This permits increased blood flow to the heart muscle, which, in turn, eases the pain from the heart.

Because heart pain tends to come on suddenly and without warning, treatment for it may require rapid administration of a drug to stop the pain. The most common form is the sublingual (under the tongue) form. Nitroglycerin tablets designed for this method of administration dissolve quickly and are absorbed into the blood circulation through the mucosa that forms the covering of the tongue and the lining of the mouth.

Many other forms of nitroglycerin are available. Some sprays may be applied under the tongue, which also provides rapid absorption. When patients have frequent or prolonged heart pain, the doctor may prescribe a long-acting oral preparation. Nitroglycerin is also made in a form that is absorbed slowly through the skin. Sometimes a paste is used for this purpose. This paste or ointment is applied directly to the skin. Another form is a patch that can be stuck directly onto the skin.

Each form of nitroglycerin has specific indications for its use. Your physician will discuss with you which form may be the most helpful for the kind of heart pain that you are experiencing.

Important Points in Therapy

If your physician has selected a nitroglycerin spray, it is used by spraying a single metered dose under the tongue. The nitroglycerin spray preparation contains about 200 doses. Unlike tablets, the spray preparation does not require refrigeration to retain potency, and it does remain stable over several years.

Notify Our Office If

- You experience chest pain.

Nitroglycerin Paste

Patient and Caregiver's Guide ■ ■ ■

General Information

Nitroglycerin has long been used in the treatment of heart pain. It causes the arterial blood vessels to widen (dilate), thereby increasing the blood flow through them to the organ that they supply. This permits increased blood flow to the heart muscle, which, in turn, eases the pain from the heart.

Nitroglycerin is made in a form that is absorbed slowly through the skin. Sometimes a paste is used for this purpose. This paste or ointment is applied directly to the skin.

Many other forms of nitroglycerin are available. If heart pain tends to come on suddenly and without warning, the treatment for it may require rapid administration of a drug to stop the pain. The most common form of nitroglycerin is the sublingual (under the tongue) form. Some sprays may be applied under the tongue, which provides rapid absorption. When patients have frequent or prolonged heart pain, the doctor may prescribe a long-acting oral preparation. Another form is a patch that can be stuck directly onto the skin.

Each form of nitroglycerin has specific indications for its use. Your physician will discuss with you which form may be most helpful for the kind of heart pain that you are experiencing.

Important Points in Therapy

If the nitroglycerin is prescribed as an ointment, it will work best if care is taken with the application to the skin. The hands and skin, in the area of application, should be clean and dry. Wash with soap and warm water, if necessary. The dose is determined by the length of ointment squeezed out of the tube. The medication will come with papers printed with a scale for this measurement. Rub the ointment over the selected area. Permit it to be absorbed. Wash your hands after application to remove any nitroglycerin that may have come off on your fingers.

189

Notify Our Office If

- You experience chest pain.
- You *do not get relief* from your chest discomfort when you use your nitroglycerin ointment.

Nitroglycerin Patches

Patient and Caregiver's Guide

General Information

Nitroglycerin has long been used in the treatment of heart pain. It causes the arterial blood vessels to widen (dilate), thereby increasing the blood flow through them to the organ that they supply. This permits increased blood flow to the heart muscle, which, in turn, eases the pain from the heart.

One form of nitroglycerin is a patch containing medication that can be stuck directly onto the skin. This is a slow-release form that is used for patients who have frequent recurrent pain.

Many other forms of nitroglycerin are available. If heart pain tends to come on suddenly and without warning, the treatment for it may require rapid administration of a drug to stop the pain. The most common form of nitroglycerin is the sublingual (under the tongue) form. Some sprays may be applied under the tongue, which provides rapid absorption. When patients have frequent or prolonged heart pain, the doctor may prescribe a long-acting oral preparation. Nitroglycerin is also made in a form that is absorbed slowly through the skin. Sometimes a paste is used for this purpose. This paste or ointment is applied directly to the skin.

Each form of nitroglycerin has specific indications for its use. Your physician will discuss with you which form may be most helpful for the kind of heart pain that you are experiencing.

Important Points in Therapy

If a nitroglycerin skin patch is prescribed, apply it only to a designated skin area. Avoid skin that is hairy. Also avoid areas that are irritated or calloused. It is wise to pick a site that will not be rubbed by clothing. The skin should be clean and dry. Wash with soap and warm water, if necessary. Handle the patch by the outside, not the sticky side, because you may rub away some of the medication. Wash your hands after application to remove any nitroglycerin that may have come off on your fingers. If you are changing patches, apply the fresh patch to a new area. This will avoid irritation of the skin.

Notify Our Office If

- You experience chest pain.
- Your nitroglycerin patch *does not give you relief* from the chest discomfort.

Atrial Flutter

General Information

Rapid heartbeat, called *tachycardia,* may have many causes. One such cause is atrial flutter. This problem occurs with increased frequency in elderly patients. It occurs with both coronary artery disease (hardening of the arteries that feed blood to the heart) and chronic bronchitis-like lung disease. Some cardiac drugs given for therapeutic purposes may alter the rhythm of the heart and produce atrial flutter as well.

The rapid heart action caused by atrial flutter is regular, with the heartbeat at 150 beats per minute. The change from a normal to a rapid rate occurs suddenly, and, often, but not always, the patient is aware of this change. Most patients can tolerate this rate change, and it poses no immediate threat to health, but the underlying problem that has caused the atrial flutter may be of great importance.

Important Points In Treatment

It is possible to restore the heart rate to normal by using drugs or, rarely, cardiac shock therapy. Prevention of atrial flutter is better than treating it. Prevention rests with adequate treatment of the underlying cause.

Notify Our Office If

- You notice a sudden change to a rapid heart rate.

Atrial Fibrillation

Patient and Caregiver's Guide

General Information

Rapid heartbeat, called *tachycardia,* may have many causes. When the heart rate and rhythm are irregular without any recognizable pattern, the problem is usually atrial fibrillation.

The heart rate and rhythm are set within the heart itself. The natural pacemaker is found within the heart. When there is a partial or complete block to the conduction of the heartbeat from this pacemaker, abnormal heart rhythms can occur. One of these abnormal heart rhythms is atrial fibrillation. In this rhythm, the normal pacemaker does not drive the heartbeat. Because the pathways are not normal, the rhythm is irregular.

This change in heart rhythm is a chronic, rather than an acute, problem. It is not the sort of rate or rhythm that changes back and forth from normal to abnormal, as occurs with many other causes of abnormal heartbeat.

Some noncardiac problems, particularly an overactive thyroid, can also cause atrial fibrillation.

Important Points In Treatment

Treatment includes the care of any underlying conditions. Medication can be used to control the heart rate by slowing the heartbeat, although the heart rhythm does not return to normal. By slowing the heartbeat, one can avoid strain on the heart and the possibility of the development of heart failure.

Because the chamber of the heart called the *atrium* may not be contracting adequately, there is a risk of the development of a blood clot, which may then break off and travel into the circulation. For this reason, some patients receive blood-thinning (anticoagulation) therapy or anti-platelet drugs, which also inhibit blood clotting.

Notify Our Office If

- You experience the onset of an *irregular* or *rapid* heart rate.

Arrhythmias

General Information

Arrhythmias are abnormalities in the rate, rhythm, or both of the heartbeat. These abnormalities occur with increasing frequency as one ages. Under normal circumstances, the heartbeat is regular in its timing, and the heart rate falls into somewhat narrow limits of numbers of heartbeats per minute. The heart rate increases with exercise.

The development of abnormal rates or rhythms has many causes. Some of these causes are primary, and others are secondary. Primary causes are those that occur within the heart. Secondary causes are those that result from external forces that act on the heart indirectly to cause a change in its rate or rhythm. It is important for your physician to separate primary from secondary causes to be able to select the most appropriate form of therapy. If the arrhythmia is secondary, it is better to treat the underlying cause than simply to try to normalize the heart rhythm with drugs and ignore what has caused the change in the first place.

Some arrhythmias pose no threat to your health. Others have great implications for the development of more serious problems. Careful evaluation to figure out the cause of the arrhythmia also permits your physician to learn the significance of the arrhythmia. The identification of the occurrence of an arrhythmia is not a dire finding, but it is an indication for further investigation.

Ordinarily, we have no perception of our own heartbeat. Irregular heart rates can come to our awareness. Single extra heartbeats may feel like "the heart turning over." Many people also notice a "racing heart" when the rate is inappropriately fast. Nonetheless, many arrhythmias occur without symptoms specific enough to alert the patient that there is abnormal heart action.

Important Points In Treatment

Treatments for arrhythmias are almost as varied as the causes of the problem itself. Arrhythmias, such as an occasional extra heartbeat, may require no therapy at all. Arrhythmias that are more persistent, that lead to the development of serious life-threatening rhythm changes, or that may cause heart failure do require treatment. Treatment may be with drugs, with the use of electronic pacemakers (devices that can be used to regulate the heart rate and rhythm), or with other devices that can alter the heart rate and rhythm.

Notify Our Office If

- You have a *frequent* or *persistent* change in your heart rate or heartbeat rhythm. The identification of an arrhythmia is not a dire finding, but it is an indication for further investigation.

Pacemakers

Patient and Caregiver's Guide

General Information

Arrhythmias are abnormalities in the rate, rhythm, or both of the heartbeat. These abnormalities occur with increasing frequency as one ages. Under normal circumstances, the heartbeat is regular in its timing, and the heart rate falls into somewhat narrow limits of numbers of heartbeats per minute. The heart rate increases with exercise.

Some arrhythmias pose no threat to your health. Others have great implications for the development of more serious problems. Careful evaluation to figure out the cause of the arrhythmia also allows your physician to determine the significance of the arrhythmia.

Many arrhythmias are treatable with medication. The best treatment for some is substituting an electronic pacemaker for the heart's own pacemaker.

Important Points In Treatment

Treatment with an electronic pacemaker (a device used to regulate the heart rate and rhythm) is used to alter the heart rate and rhythm and keep the heart rate close to normal. If this therapy is done for a very short time in the hospital, a pacemaker device outside the body is connected by wires to the heart muscle. This is a temporary pacemaker. If longer-term treatment is necessary, a tiny battery-powered pacemaker may be placed under the skin by a surgeon. These are implanted pacemakers.

Implanting a pacemaker is not a major operation. Some restrictions on activity are necessary for 4 to 6 weeks after pacemaker insertion. Until the healing of the incision and around the wires to the heart is complete, you should not do heavy lifting, arm exercises, or stretching with the arm on the pacemaker side of the body. Often a loose sling is worn as a reminder. This arm should be kept active, but without strain. Controlled activity is important to prevent the joints from stiffening and the arm from becoming weak. Often you must learn to slip loose clothes, such as a sweatshirt, over the pacemaker-side arm and shoulder first when dressing.

Pacemakers require regular checkups and service. With regular maintenance, they can last for 10 years or more before replacement. Pacemaker checkups require only a brief visit to the physician. Sometimes physicians have equipment that allows these checkups to be done over the telephone. Besides these checkups by your physician, it is important and prudent to monitor the pacemaker function yourself on a daily basis. The pacemaker keeps your pulse at a set rate. Some pacemakers increase the rate automatically when you exercise, but at rest they return to the set rate. If you take your pulse rate each day at rest and at approximately the same time, you should have the same heart rate. If this rate varies or if there is any irregularity of the rhythm, you must notify your physician.

Carry a pacemaker identification card so that, in case of an accident or serious illness, those attending to you are aware of the existence of your pacemaker. Pacemakers are well shielded from electrical interference from the outside, but electrical currents and microwaves can affect them.

Occasionally, a patient will feel fatigue or dizziness. Fainting may occur. It is also possible to experience a feeling of pulsation in the neck or in the chest. If this occurs, it is a sign that the pacemaker needs adjustment.

 ## Notify Our Office If

- You have a *frequent* or *persistent* change in your heart rate or heartbeat rhythm.
- You have any sign of *inflammation, heat, tenderness,* or *swelling* around the pacemaker.
- You experience unexplained *fatigue, dizziness,* or *fainting* or if there is a sensation of *pulsation* in your neck or chest.

Implantable Cardioverter-Defibrillators

Patient and Caregiver's Guide ■ ■ ■

General Information

In patients with a prior history of serious cardiac arrhythmias or a sudden stopping of the heartbeat, an implantable cardioverter may be recommended. This is a device that automatically provides an electric charge to the heart, like an external defibrillator, when it senses a critical change in the heart rate or rhythm.

Implanting a cardioverter is not a major operation. Some restrictions on activity are necessary for 4 to 6 weeks after pacemaker insertion. Until the healing of the incision and around the wires to the heart is complete, you should not do heavy lifting, arm exercises, or stretching with the arm on the pacemaker side of the body. Often a loose sling is worn as a reminder. This arm should be kept active but without strain. Controlled activity is important to prevent the joints from stiffening and the arm from becoming weak. Often you must learn to slip loose clothes, such as a sweatshirt, over the cardioverter-side arm and shoulder first when dressing.

Cardioverters require regular checkups and service. With regular maintenance, they can last for 10 years or more before replacement. Cardioverter checkups require only a brief visit to the physician. Sometimes physicians have equipment that allows these checkups to be done over the telephone. Besides these checkups by your physician, it is important and prudent to monitor the pacemaker function yourself on a daily basis. The pacemaker keeps your pulse at a set rate. Some pacemakers increase the rate automatically when you exercise, but at rest they return to the set rate. If you take your pulse rate each day at rest and at approximately the same time, you should have the same heart rate. If this rate varies or if there is any irregularity of the rhythm, you must notify your physician.

Carry a cardioverter identification card so that in case of an accident or serious illness, those attending to you are aware of the existence of your cardioverter. Cardioverters are well shielded from electrical interference from the outside, but electrical currents and microwaves can affect them. Usually the device can be felt in its pocket underneath the skin. One should avoid twisting the device. Such twisting may cause the connections with the heart to be interrupted.

The doctor may suggest a short interval of restriction in driving an automobile following the implantation of the defibrillator. There is a small risk that triggering the cardioverter may cause temporary impairment in the ability to drive, resulting in an accident. As indicated, this restriction is usually temporary. Once the patient's tolerance of the defibrillator has been observed, the restriction would be lifted. On average this observation takes about 6 months.

 ## Notify Our Office If

- You have a *frequent* or *persistent* triggering of your defibrillator.
- You have any sign of *inflammation, heat, tenderness,* or *swelling* around the pacemaker.
- You experience unexplained *fatigue, dizziness,* or *fainting* or if there is a sensation of *pulsation* in your neck or chest.

Heart Failure

Patient and Caregiver's Guide

General Information

Heart failure occurs when, for whatever reason, the heart is unable to pump sufficient blood to meet the body's needs. Heart failure has many possible causes, and it may occur at any age from infancy on, but the prevalence of heart failure clearly increases after age 60.

Careful diagnosis of the cause or causes of the heart failure offers the best opportunity for treatment. The signs and symptoms are much the same with any of the various causes of heart failure. Elderly patients may not have typical symptoms. Fatigue, sleeplessness, disorientation, and confusion are early signs of heart failure in elderly patients. Vascular changes may be noted in the legs and feet. Weakness is often present. The common symptoms of heart failure do occur in elderly patients, but often they are not the earliest signs and symptoms.

Important Points In Treatment

Specific treatment for heart failure depends on its cause. When your doctor can find a cause that can be treated directly, it will be treated. Anemia, high blood pressure, and hyperthyroidism are a few of these causes. A number of blood tests not directly related to the heart may be performed to search for causes. If a specific cause cannot be found or cannot be adequately treated, medications directed at the heart failure will be used. Five kinds of drugs are used to treat patients with heart failure: digitalis, diuretics, ACE inhibitors, beta blockers, and vasodilators.

1. Digitalis, which is the traditional drug for the treatment of heart failure, improves the heart's function as a pump. Careful control of the dosage is necessary to get a full effect without producing complicating side effects. Some patients' problems do not warrant or require the use of digitalis.

2. Diuretics are drugs that promote the output of excess fluid. Decreasing the fluid accumulation decreases the amount of

work the heart must do as a pump and thus lessens the severity of the heart failure. Often, potassium supplements are necessary to avoid losses that may accompany the use of diuretic drugs.

3. Vasodilator drugs relax the blood vessels. These drugs, by decreasing muscular contraction of the blood vessels, may also decrease the work that the heart must perform as a pump. This may improve the circumstances of the heart failure.

4. ACE inhibitors are drugs that modify the pressures within the blood vessels. These drugs can reduce the strain under which the heart is placed.

5. Beta blockers are drugs that will slow the heart rate and thus reduce the strain on the heart. These drugs have side effects and require careful dosing.

Besides these specific drugs, several measures that improve heart function do not involve medications. Adequate daily rest interspersed with mild exercise, such as walking, can help you prevent edema and retain physical fitness. Your physician will help you find the limits of exercise that are appropriate in light of your heart disease. Limitation of dietary salt may also help control fluid accumulation and improve heart function. The stringency of salt restriction depends on the kind of drugs you are given and your customary salt intake. Generally, a dietitian tailors the amount of salt restriction to the needs of the individual patient, and your physician will help you with this determination.

If you are overweight, a careful program of weight reduction may also help restore heart function. Avoid exposure to extremes of heat and cold, which call upon an extra measure of heart function to help you remain comfortable.

Notify Our Office If

- You develop unusual fatigue or shortness of breath, awaken at night short of breath, or notice persistent ankle swelling. These symptoms are often found with heart failure.
- You experience minor changes in behavior, activity, or mentation. Elderly patients may have less-typical symptoms, and often the symptoms are of a less-specific character.

Myocardial Infarction

Patient and Caregiver's Guide

General Information

When the circulation of blood through the coronary arteries—the arteries that feed blood to the heart muscle—decreases too much, a portion of the heart muscle dies. This is a myocardial infarction, or a *heart attack*. Hardening of the coronary arteries occurs because of the deposition of cholesterol in the walls of the blood vessels. These deposits prevent the blood vessel from relaxing and opening wider when necessary, and they may also narrow the existing opening in the blood vessel, thereby impairing the flow of blood. The surface of these narrowed cholesterol-filled areas may become covered by a blood clot that stops the blood flow. Any of these changes may produce a myocardial infarction.

A heart attack is a life-threatening illness. If the amount of heart muscle that dies is large, the heart will be unable to pump enough blood to sustain the body's needs, and death occurs. Even if the amount of muscle lost is small enough to permit the heart to continue to serve as an adequate pump, there is the danger that the weakened heart wall may rupture or that damage has occurred to the heart's conduction system, either of which may also result in death. Blood clots may form on the damaged heart wall, and, if they break free, the clots can enter the circulation and cause damage where they finally lodge. The heart may be so crippled as a pump that there is limitation of other physical activity.

The most common sign of a heart attack is chest pain. This is most often felt in the front of the left side of the chest. Additional pain may be felt in the neck, jaw, left shoulder or left arm, or back. Less commonly, pain may be felt in the abdomen. The pain may mimic gallbladder disease, ulcers, or heartburn. As the severity of the heart damage increases, other symptoms and signs may appear. If there is beginning heart failure, breathlessness will be prominent. The heart may race unusually fast or become abnormally slow. With heart failure there is weakness, and swelling of the lower legs may develop.

Important Points In Treatment

A myocardial infarction is always an indication for hospitalization. Where such facilities are available, patients are placed in specialized areas called *coronary care units*. This allows the patient to have continuous monitoring of the heart rate and rhythm. The trained nursing personnel in coronary care units have the resources to do cardiac resuscitation.

Early in the course of a myocardial infarction, it may be possible to dissolve the clot, saving much of the affected muscle. Often this is done in conjunction with an emergency cardiac catheterization. In addition, the use of other drugs, such as aspirin, may limit the extent of the damage to the heart muscle. Rapid access to medical help is necessary for many of these interventions.

Rehabilitation after a heart attack is important to support the patient in regaining the maximal level of activity. Other measures can be taken to lessen the likelihood of a second heart attack. Exercising, reducing blood cholesterol and other fats, and stopping smoking are important parts of this rehabilitation.

Notify Our Office If

- You have sudden onset of chest pain. *This is a medical emergency*. A heart attack is a life-threatening illness. If the amount of heart muscle that dies is large, the heart will fail to pump enough blood to sustain the body's needs, and death will occur.

Cardiovascular Rehabilitation

Patient and Caregiver's Guide ▪ ▪ ▪

 ## General Information

Many patients undertake a cardiac rehabilitation program after a heart attack, after surgery on the heart or its arteries, and sometimes after insertion of supports called *stents* into narrowed arteries after they're stretching (dilatation) or just stretching of the arteries in the heart. The program involves both exercise and education to help patients return to the most active and productive life that they can achieve. In the past, failure to undertake cardiac rehabilitation has caused some patients to suffer unnecessary limitations of lifestyle.

Cardiac rehabilitation must be set for each individual patient's needs. Usually, some tests are performed to help the therapist determine, with your physician, which components of cardiac rehabilitation are most suitable and where to begin. These tests include a cardiac stress test, a determination of blood fats (including cholesterol), and a dietary history.

The exercise component of rehabilitation begins with exercise directed toward the highest level of heart activity that you can safely tolerate. Riding a stationary bicycle and stair climbing are commonly used exercises. The therapist monitors the heart rate and blood pressure to ensure that exercise is kept within safe limits. As your body and heart permit, the therapist increases this level of exercise gradually. The ideal goal is to restore you to a functioning level at or above level before illness.

The education component of rehabilitation addresses all of the other risk factors associated with the development and progression of heart disease. These include weight reduction, stopping smoking, and proper blood pressure control. If your blood tests or diet history suggests that it is helpful, there is instruction in the selection and preparation of foods to lower cholesterol and salt in the diet.

Notify Our Office If

- You have onset of any kind of discomfort or pain in the chest.
- You experience any shortness of breath or ankle swelling.
- Your exercise causes any discomfort in your bones or joints.

Antibiotic Prophylaxis in Patients with Heart Disease

Patient and Caregiver's Guide

General Information

Many patients with heart disease, particularly those who have had cardiac surgery with replacement valves, may be unusually susceptible to bacterial infection involving the heart. They are at risk when they have other medical or dental procedures, which can cause a shower of bacteria into the blood, possibly causing an infection in the heart. Not all patients with heart disease are susceptible to these kinds of infections.

Antibiotic prophylaxis is indicated in patients who have a prior history of infection in the heart and in those who have had replacement heart valves inserted at surgery. In addition, some patients with congenital heart disease and patients who have had surgery to fashion connections between the chambers of the heart or large vessels are also susceptible. These patients should receive antibiotic prophylaxis when a procedure that can cause bacteria to enter the circulation is planned.

In addition, some patients with acquired disease of the heart valves, some heart muscle diseases called *cardiomyopathy* and *mitral valve prolapse* associated with changes in the blood flow are at moderate risk for developing infection. These patients usually receive antibiotic prophylaxis as well.

Important Points in Therapy

Be sure that you inform any physician or dentist of your cardiac problems at the time they suggest any sort of medical or dental procedure. In addition, they must know whether you have an allergy to any of the antibiotics.

Notify Our Office If

- You are planning to undergo a medical, surgical, or dental procedure.

Aortic Aneurysm

Patient and Caregiver's Guide

General Information

An *aneurysm* is an abnormal dilatation (enlargement) in an artery. The dilatation occurs because of a weakness in the wall of the artery. These weak areas are subject to rupture, with disastrous consequences. Besides rupturing, these enlargements may cause pressure on other organs or on nerves, or they may develop a clot, called a *thrombosis*. The risk of the aneurysm varies with its location and the likelihood that it may rupture. Size is an indication of the likelihood of rupture. Larger aneurysms are at greater risk of rupture.

Aneurysms occur with increased frequency in elderly patients. The changes in arterial blood vessels that occur with aging permit the development of areas of weakness that ultimately become aneurysms. Aneurysms tend to be more likely in individuals with high blood pressure *that remains uncontrolled*. Aneurysms do occur in younger patients, but these are often the result of an abnormality present in the artery from birth, although a few of these may remain undetected until later years.

In elderly patients, the most common aneurysm is in the aorta, the large artery carrying blood directly from the heart to the abdomen and legs. An aneurysm in this location usually causes no symptoms, so it remains silent until rupture occurs or is pending. Because the risk for rupture is high, there is interest in repairing the damaged blood vessel by removing the weakened section and replacing it with a graft. Aneurysms may occur in the aorta as it passes through the chest and in the larger branches of the aorta. These, too, pose some risk, but a surgically placed graft (replacement for the vessel) can repair the weakness.

Another form of aortic aneurysm that occurs with increased frequency in elderly patients is the dissecting aneurysm. A small tear occurs in the lining of the aorta, and blood may spread up and down within the wall of the blood vessel. As this happens, the blood in the wall of the aorta may partially or completely occlude the openings of the blood vessels that branch off the aorta. This can cause stroke, loss of kidney function, or symptoms of vascular insufficiency in the limbs or other organs. *Dissecting aneurysm is an emergency* that usually requires treatment with surgery.

Aneurysms involving the aorta are often easily identified by an ultrasound examination. This test is simple, painless, and noninvasive. It can identify the otherwise silent aneurysmal dilatations that occur in the aorta and some of the large arteries.

Notify Our Office If

- You feel a lump that throbs in time with your heartbeat. The risk of the aneurysm varies with its location and the likelihood that it may rupture.
- You experience sudden chest pain that does not subside. Dissecting aneurysm is an emergency that usually requires treatment with surgery.

Primary Varicose Veins

Patient and Caregiver's Guide ■ ■ ■

General Information

Varicose veins are dilated (enlarged) superficial veins. They can occur in any area of the body surface, but they are primarily a problem in the legs. There are several causes for the dilatation that occurs in superficial veins. Primary varicose veins are a result of gradual degeneration in the valves within the veins. These valves occur at regular intervals along the course of the veins. The valves permit blood to flow toward the heart and restrict the ability of blood to flow away from the heart and into the veins. These valves prevent the development of high pressure within leg veins even when one is standing.

The tendency toward valvular degeneration is familial. Primary varicose veins cause little, if any, interference in the health of the individual, but they do gradually increase in frequency with age. Three fourths of the population of the United States age 65 or older have varicose veins.

The development of varicose veins occurs earlier in those individuals destined to develop valvular degeneration, particularly if they wear garments that permit blockage of the flow of blood in the veins. Constricting bands from elastic garments, garters, and hose (particularly hose with elastic leg bands) cause slowing of the blood flow in veins below the point of constriction. Careful attention to unimpeded venous blood flow can delay the onset of varicose veins and slow their progression, even in patients who by familial history are unusually susceptible.

Important Points In Treatment

Most of the concern related to primary varicose veins is related to appearance. Occasionally, a varicose vein may be traumatized and bleed or develop clots and become inflamed, but these are infrequent complications. Complications of this sort tend to not be life threatening.

Treatment involves the use of support hose. Such hose must be well fitting and provide firm, even support over the entire leg. If you wear ill-fitting support stockings, they will permit periodic constriction that leads to worsening of the varicose veins rather than their prevention. Support garments often need to be tailor-made to provide satisfactory relief.

Surgical procedures strip out the distended veins or obliterate them by injection. Obtaining the guidance of your physician is wise when determining the desirability of undergoing such procedures solely for cosmetic reasons.

Your physician may use one of several diagnostic methods to distinguish primary varicose veins from secondary varicose veins. This is important because treatment opportunities are different for each variety. Secondary varicose veins are a result of damage to deep veins. The deep venous insufficiency may be related to dire complications and requires careful management.

Notify Our Office If

- You have a varicose vein that becomes *red, hard,* or *tender.*
- You have a varicose vein that begins to bleed.

Secondary Varicose Veins

Patient and Caregiver's Guide

General Information

Varicose veins are dilated (enlarged) superficial veins. They can occur in any area of the body surface, but they are primarily a problem of the legs. There are several causes for the dilatation that occurs in superficial veins. Secondary varicose veins are distended superficial veins that form because of insufficiency in the deeper leg veins. Deep vein insufficiency is a result of thrombophlebitis, inflammation, and deterioration involving the deep veins. The obstruction of the veins and the associated inflammation cause impairment of the valves in the veins. This results in unusual pressure on the superficial veins that are just beneath the skin. These superficial veins become distended with blood and are visible as tortuous veins beneath the skin.

The superficial veins are an unfortunate cosmetic consequence of serious disease in the deeper veins. The visible varicose veins themselves pose little health risk.

Important Points In Treatment

It is most important to treat the deep vein thrombophlebitis and to prevent the chronic deep venous insufficiency that is a result. Reduction of inflammation and of chronic edema not only prevents further complications of deep venous insufficiency but also can slow and arrest or even prevent the development of superficial varicose veins. During acute attacks of thrombophlebitis, anti-coagulants (blood-thinning agents) are often needed. As chronic insufficiency develops, attention moves to preventing edema. Elevation of the legs several times daily can help keep swelling down, as can the use of properly fitting support hose. Poorly fitting hose may result in the development of worsening deep vein thrombosis. Other garments that may be tight or restrictive around the leg or thigh should be avoided as well.

Notify Our Office If

- You notice *swelling* and *tenderness* or *redness* in your calf.

Air Travel Phlebitis

Patient and Caregiver's Guide

General Information

Prolonged immobilization may lead to the slowing of blood flow in the legs and can permit the formation of blood clots. This can occur with bed rest, but it can also occur with prolonged periods of sitting that are common with travel. Automobile travel, rail travel, and airline travel have all been associated with the development of these blood clots, a condition called *phlebitis.*

Other factors besides immobilization may be a part of the problem. Dehydration is one of these factors. Patients with heart or kidney problems that predispose them to developing edema or swelling of the legs may also be susceptible to this problem.

Important Points In Treatment

If you are going to take a trip that requires prolonged immobilization, attempt to maintain your hydration and, if possible, to break the trip at regular intervals to permit brief exercise. Even while confined in an airline seat, it is possible to exercise the lower legs and feet while sitting still. Any airlines offer on their entertainment channels programs of this sort.

Notify Our Office If

- You develop redness or swelling in your lower leg after prolonged sitting during travel.

Edema of the Legs (Dropsy)

Patient and Caregiver's Guide

General Information

Swelling of the lower legs is common at any age and even more so in older people. Edema of this sort, called *dropsy,* occurs with heart failure, but many other possible causes exist besides failing heart function. Many of these causes are temporary and are not life threatening. A few herald more serious health problems or can lead to complications that can be serious and disabling.

Edema represents the accumulation of excess fluid in the tissues but outside the arteries and veins. The most common cause of edema is gravity.

Some tissue fluid is present in all of us. The system that removes this fluid and returns it to the blood circulation is able to just keep up with fluid formation under ordinary circumstances and at usual levels of activity. This system depends, in part, on the muscular contraction of the leg muscles against the veins and the tissue spaces to help pump this tissue fluid back into the circulatory system. If there are limits on exercise and mobility, excess fluid can accumulate by gravity in the lowermost portion of the body. Physicians often speak of this as *dependent edema* because it goes to the most dependent (lowest) portions of the body.

This is really the familiar story that all of us have experienced when taking a long automobile or airplane trip. With this prolonged inactivity, enough swelling of the feet and ankles develops to prevent our getting our shoes back on after the trip. With the resumption of activity, this accumulation of fluid rapidly resolves, and the edema disappears. In elderly patients who are bedridden or chair-bound for long periods, this edema can worsen. It can develop to the point at which there is sufficient swelling to lead to secondary complications.

Important Points In Treatment

Changes in position, particularly elevation of the feet, can move this fluid accumulation and lessen the possibility of complications. Often, when the fluid moves, it may find a location where the edema is less apparent, but the fluid accumulation remains. This is particularly true in people who lie down without turning over for long periods. Fluid that may have accumulated in the legs while they were sitting or standing flows into the back. With the distribution over a larger area, the edema is somewhat less apparent. The fluid nonetheless continues to be present. It is better to promote the removal of the fluid than it is to shift the fluid from one area to another.

Even limited exercise can resolve the edema. Your tolerance for exercise plus the guidance of your physician will help establish safe limits for exercise. Although levels of exercise to acquire physical fitness may need to be extreme, those necessary to promote the removal of edema fluid may be much less strenuous.

If there is only limited opportunity for exercise, your physician may add the use of diuretic drugs and restriction of salt (sodium) intake to help limit the formation of edema. Overtreatment can occur, leading to kidney dysfunction. Therefore, the use of diuretic drugs must be carefully controlled. Indiscriminate use may precipitate complications.

In addition to the use of diet and drugs, the use of support stockings or hose can help restrict the accumulation of fluid in the legs. These must be carefully fitted and continually adjusted to prevent complications that can be associated with tight-fitting garments.

Heart disease and liver disease may also cause edema. Heart failure is a well-recognized cause of edema and is commonly the first thing that comes to a physician's mind when an individual has swollen legs. Treatment involves improvement of heart function to permit it to work more effectively as a pump, with modifications in salt and water intake to reduce the load on the heart. Impaired liver function may change the blood composition enough to cause the accumulation of tissue fluids. Certain drugs, particularly steroids and reproductive hormones, may also be associated with fluid retention.

Varicose veins and other forms of peripheral vascular disease that cause an impediment to good venous circulation may permit the accumulation of tissue fluids more rapidly than they can be carried back into the circulation. Many individuals have had thrombophlebitis (inflammation in the veins) and impairment of their circulation. Because of this inflammation, they have a residual problem of the easy accumulation of edema fluid.

These problems can be cumulative. In elderly patients in whom heart failure, minimal venous slowing, and inactivity may all occur, the combination of these effects may result in the production of prolonged edema even though each individual problem might not be serious enough to cause edema on its own.

Leg and ankle swelling may be caused by problems other than simple fluid accumulation. Infections of the legs or feet cause swelling, just as infections anywhere in the body do. It is also possible for fractures or cracks to appear in bones subjected to unusual stress. These silent fractures may also cause tissue swelling to occur.

Notify Our Office If

- You have swelling or edema in the legs or ankles. Report the occurrence of swelling of the legs when you visit your physician.

Hypertension

Patient and Caregiver's Guide ▪ ▪ ▪

General Information

Hypertension is the sustained elevation of blood pressure above normal levels. It is a common occurrence in the elderly, but it is not a consequence of the aging process. It has many possible causes. Not all are known. On occasion, for brief intervals, there may be elevations in blood pressure that are not part of hypertension.

Clearly, sustained elevation of blood pressure may lead to heart disease, stroke, and kidney failure. Treatment to lower blood pressure to normal levels reduces these risks even in elderly patients.

The measurement of blood pressure with the commonly used blood pressure cuff involves many possible sources of error. Physicians are unlikely to make a diagnosis of hypertension from one or even several blood pressure measurements, unless the pressures measured are very high. They may ask you to return for repeated blood pressure checks for several days to determine whether you have true sustained high blood pressure.

Important Points In Treatment

If a cause for the elevated blood pressure can be found, it is best to try to lower the pressure to normal by treating the cause. In many patients no cause can be found (this is essential hypertension), and in some people treatment of the cause might have begun too late to permit the blood pressure to return to normal. Your physician may choose to start treatment to lower your blood pressure directly.

Besides drugs, other forms of treatment are effective in reducing blood pressure in some patients. These include weight loss, exercise, stopping smoking, low-salt diet, calcium supplements, and stress management. These other forms of therapy may not be completely successful in lowering your blood pressure to normal, but they can reduce the amount of medication needed and thus reduce the possibility or severity of drug-related side effects.

Many kinds of blood pressure–reducing drugs are available. These include diuretics, vasodilators, adrenergic inhibitors, calcium channel–blocking drugs, and enzyme inhibitors (ACE inhibitors). You may hear from family or friends that they know of someone taking one or several of these different classes of drugs. The selection of the proper drug depends on your degree of high blood pressure and on your other medical problems. Some of the medications used to treat high blood pressure can bring out or worsen other diseases. The selection of the drug and the dosage are individualized for each patient.

The treatment of high blood pressure often involves a complex program that includes several elements. Do not hesitate to discuss the program with your physician so that you understand the function of each element in your antihypertension program, lest an important element be omitted.

Changes in blood pressure with treatment occur slowly. Rapid changes may be harmful or cause side effects. In some patients, careful monitoring of blood pressure at home with a blood pressure cuff is helpful. You should be aware that there may be differences in the blood pressure measured by different observers using different cuffs. It is best to have blood pressure checks done at the same location. Coin-operated blood pressure cuffs found in stores are notoriously inaccurate and are not reliable to monitor blood pressure.

Postural Hypotension

Patient and Caregiver's Guide

General Information

Postural hypotension, which physicians also call *orthostatic hypotension,* is a fall in the blood pressure that occurs when one goes from a lying to a standing position. This fall in blood pressure when rising can cause weakness, light-headedness, dizziness, or syncope (fainting). It is a problem that emerges with increasing frequency with advancing age.

There are multiple causes. Vascular and nervous system changes with age can, alone, produce this reaction in the blood pressure. Diseases that affect the cardiovascular system and the nervous system can do so as well. A number of endocrine diseases can also be involved. Many drugs may produce this response as an effect or a side effect.

Your doctor will undertake a comprehensive review of your medical history and physical examination to look for possible causes. A number of laboratory and other tests may be required to identify or eliminate possible causes.

Important Points In Treatment

The best treatment is prevention. When the underlying cause is identified, it should be treated. When the cause remains obscure or the treatment is not adequate to relieve the symptoms of the orthostatic hypotension, some general measures are helpful. These include but are not limited to:

1. Avoid bed rest during the daytime. Sitting rather than reclining may lessen the postural effect.
2. Elevate the head of the bed on 6-inch blocks. This will lessen the fluid shifts usually experienced when lying down.
3. When you rise from the bed, sit up first and wait several minutes before standing.
4. Some patients benefit from putting on support stockings before rising to a standing position.
5. Your doctor may advise you about the addition of salt to your diet.

Notify Our Office If

- You begin to experience dizziness or light-headedness on rising to a standing position.
- You faint.

Beta Blockers

Patient and Caregiver's Guide

General Information

The drugs called *beta blockers* are widely used for the treatment of a variety of conditions that are common in the elderly. They have an effect on the heart rate and on the blood vessels. They are extensively used for angina (heart pain), after heart attacks, for high blood pressure, and for heart failure. These drugs are also used for the prevention of migraine headaches, for the treatment of some kinds of anxiety, for parkinsonism, and in some patients with liver trouble.

These drugs have a wide variety of effects and side effects and should be taken only under the direction and observation of your physician.

Important Points in Therapy

One of the direct effects of these drugs is the slowing of the heart rate. This means that your heart rate will not rise as high or as fast with exercise. This may cause some slight limitation of the speed and endurance with which you can approach tasks. Usually, with exercise your heart rate rises to supply blood to working muscles. Without enough blood flow, the muscles will fatigue quickly. There must then be a brief interval of rest to permit the blood flow to catch up with the muscles' metabolic needs. The rest needed may only be a matter of a half a minute or less before you are ready to continue your tasks.

The drug should not be stopped abruptly. It may require a graduated discontinuance of the medicine to avoid the recurrence of symptoms.

This class of drug will interact with many other medications. Be sure to tell your physician about all of the medications that you are taking, including nonprescription drugs and drugs that you take only occasionally.

Side effects of the drugs may involve many bodily systems. Side effects do not occur in all patients. Cardiac side effects may include a very slow heart rate and postural (orthostatic) hypotension. Some men suffer impotence. Asthma-like bronchospasm will occur in a few patients. The drug may have effects on the central nervous system, including depression, confusion, insomnia, and dizziness. These usually happen when the drug is first started or the dose is changed. Careful follow-up with your physician is necessary to ensure that you are receiving the proper dose to get the full benefit with minimum or no side effects.

Notify Our Office If

- You experience any of the above-mentioned side effects while taking a beta blocker drug.
- You decide that you must *stop* taking the drug for any reason.

Cardiac Catheterization

Patient and Caregiver's Guide ■ ■ ■

 ## General Information

A cardiac catheterization is a procedure in which the physician passes a long, thin tube through a blood vessel into your heart. This tube, called a *catheter,* may be introduced through a vein or through an artery. Sometimes vessels in the leg are used, and sometimes those in the arm are used. The type and location of the vessel used vary with the information that is needed.

Through this catheter the physician can measure pressures in the heart chamber and across the heart valves. It is also possible to measure the oxygen content of the blood in the various locations. It is possible to inject dye into the heart chambers and vessels that will show on x-rays. This permits the identification of abnormal openings or blockages in the heart or its blood vessels. It is also possible to measure the electrical activity of portions of the heart, which can be important in patients who have difficulty maintaining a normal heart rate or rhythm.

Often it is possible for the physician to use the catheter to open blocked areas or to perform other adjustments to the heart without the need for an open surgical operation.

PREPARATION FOR THE EXAMINATION

Usually, you will be asked to avoid eating from midnight the night before the examination. Be sure to tell the physician if you have an allergy to any medications or to the dye used for x-ray films. If you have difficulty lying flat on your back for a prolonged time, tell this to the physician. If you have been taking blood-thinning drugs, aspirin, or aspirin-like drugs, tell the physician. The physician may ask other questions about your medical history.

After the procedure, its alternatives, its objectives, and its complications have been explained to you, you will be asked to sign a consent for the performance of this procedure. If you have any questions concerning this information or the procedure itself, ask the doctor before signing the consent form. The doctor will be willing to try to answer all of your questions.

DURING THE CATHETERIZATION

You may be given some premedication before the examination. Often the locations of your pulse in different areas will be marked to help when the time comes to pass the catheter. In addition to one or two physicians, other assistants and nurses may be in the room.

The catheterization will be performed on a special table with x-ray available. An intravenous line will be started. The area where the catheter will be introduced will be shaved and cleaned (prepped). A local anesthetic will be injected into this area.

After the catheter is introduced into the blood vessel, it will be threaded under x-ray guidance into the selected areas of the heart. At various times, dye may be injected to obtain x-ray images of the heart chambers or blood vessels. When this happens, you will be warned. You may feel a warm flush and/or some chest discomfort.

AFTER THE PROCEDURE

The whole procedure usually takes 1 or 1.5 hours. When the catheter is removed, bleeding from that spot will be controlled with pressure. You will then be taken to a recovery area and later to your hospital room. If the catheter was passed through blood vessels in the groin, you will have a pressure bandage and will need to lie flat with your legs straight. If you need to urinate or move your bowels, you must use a bedpan. If a blood vessel in your wrist or arm was used, it will have a pressure dressing, but you will be able to sit up and to use the bathroom. You may be asked to wear a sling and to not use the arm for several days. It is wise to have loose fitting clothes and button-front shirts to wear home.

The results from the procedure are usually available very shortly after its completion. Because of the medication you receive, the doctor may delay discussing these results until you have recovered and are fully awake.

Notify Our Office If

- You notice any bleeding from the area where the catheter was passed into the blood vessel.
- You have a hand or foot that becomes cold or numb or has pins-and-needles sensations.
- You experience chest discomfort or shortness of breath.
- You become dizzy or light-headed.
- You develop a skin rash.

CHAPTER 10

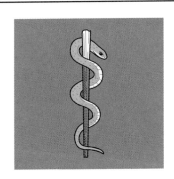
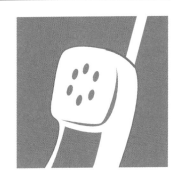

Pulmonary Problems

Emphysema

Patient and Caregiver's Guide

General Information

Chronic pulmonary (lung) disease, often called *chronic obstructive pulmonary disease* or COPD, usually involves a combination of chronic bronchitis and emphysema. Inflammation in the large air passages in the lungs causes chronic bronchitis, which, in turn, causes persistent irritation. The result is chronic cough with sputum production that generally occurs for 3 or more months of the year.

Emphysema is a condition of enlarged or overdistended air sacs in the lung. The air sacs are enlarged at the expense of lung tissue. There is less lung to breathe with, and this distortion makes breathing with the remaining lung less efficient. When emphysema occurs with chronic bronchitis, the disease may become severe enough for patients to suffer respiratory insufficiency (lung failure).

Emphysema is a result of breathing in irritants. In addition, many patients inherit a predisposition to the development of emphysema. Avoiding the inhalation of irritants can prevent or delay the development of emphysema. In patients already affected, avoidance of irritants can slow or arrest the progress of the disease.

Important Points In Treatment

The first and most prevalent irritant to avoid is cigarette smoke. In some areas, exposure to high levels of air pollution is an additional problem. Relocation is a solution, but this may not be possible for all. Maintaining a dust-free room and using filters with forced-air heating or air-conditioning systems can provide a bridge to survive difficult days. Air filtration systems can remove large and small particles from the air and may be a useful adjunct in maintaining a dust-free room. Prevention of influenza and pneumonia with vaccine, as well as careful treatment of upper respiratory tract infections and flu with adequate fluids, can prevent crippling and life-threatening lung infections.

As emphysema progresses, respiratory therapy may be needed to promote drainage from the lungs and to keep the airways clean. Respiratory therapy can also supplement the oxygen supply. Respiratory failure and the effort of breathing may cause weakness and impose restrictions on activity. A creative approach is necessary to perform the daily tasks of living. Regulate your activities to avoid exposure to respiratory insults. Adjust your environment and your diet to simplify the tasks of daily living. Preserve your independence.

Notify Our Office If

- You have *any sign* of respiratory tract infection. Seek medical help from your physician at the first sign of respiratory tract infection.
- You are interested in stopping smoking. There are many approaches now available for smoking cessation. Not every program is suitable for every patient. We can help you to decide which program might best fit your needs.

Chronic Bronchitis

Patient and Caregiver's Guide

General Information

Chronic pulmonary (lung) disease, often called *chronic obstructive pulmonary disease* or COPD, usually involves a combination of chronic bronchitis and emphysema. Inflammation in the large air passages in the lungs causes chronic bronchitis, which, in turn, causes persistent irritation. The result is chronic cough with sputum production that generally occurs for 3 or more months of the year.

The changes in the airways in the lungs that occur with chronic bronchitis are a result of exposure to airborne irritants plus recurrent and chronic infections in the bronchi. The most common of these irritants is cigarette smoke, but there are many occupational exposures, as well as exposures to airborne pollutants in the environment.

The chronic irritation that results can increase the secretion of mucus in the lungs. There is difficulty in clearing the excess secretions, and this may add to the development of emphysema.

Important Points In Treatment

Management includes the use of adequate fluids and humidity to help you cough up excess secretions. Your physician may prescribe medications to help thin these secretions. Take care to avoid lung irritants. You must also take extraordinary care to avoid and, if necessary, to obtain treatment for upper respiratory tract infections and influenza. Patients with chronic bronchitis are much more susceptible to secondary infection, complicating colds or flu and perhaps causing pneumonia. Vaccination and careful, prudent personal hygiene are in order, but these preventives are not perfect. Report even minor respiratory tract infections to your physician promptly for treatment and sometimes to receive prophylaxis to prevent the development of pneumonia.

231

Notify Our Office If

- You have *any sign* of respiratory tract infection. Seek medical help from your physician at the first sign of respiratory tract infection.
- You are interested in stopping smoking. Many approaches are now available for smoking cessation. Not every program is suitable for every patient. We can help you decide which program might best fit your needs.

Asthma

Patient and Caregiver's Guide

General Information

Asthma is a disease that causes a breathing problem. Individuals with asthma develop an obstruction to breathing in the very small airways in the lung, called *bronchi*. This obstruction is usually reversible, although it may be only partially reversible in the advanced stage of the disease. There frequently is associated inflammation in the air passages. The air passages become very sensitive to a variety of stimuli. The older concept of asthma representing an allergy to elements in the air is not completely true. Other sorts of stimuli can also precipitate asthmatic attacks.

Three symptoms that are commonly present in asthmatic attacks are wheezing, cough, and chronic shortness of breath. All three of these elements do not need to be present for a diagnosis of asthma.

Although asthmatic attacks may cause serious disability, the attack itself is usually not cause of death unless other complicating features occur. Careful treatment may help avoid these complicating features.

Important Points in Therapy

Patients with a diagnosis of asthma usually have a need for monitoring of lung function. An attempt is made to eliminate or control those particular factors in any individual patient that seem to act as triggers for asthmatic attacks. This includes being sure that the patient is immunized against pneumonia and influenza. There is also a need to alter the environment to reduce or eliminate triggering factors. An example would be problems brought on by exposure to pets.

It may be important to attempt to provide a dust-free environment, at least a dust-free room, as a retreat from environmental triggers. It is also possible to use some medications in anticipation of an inevitable exposure to a trigger.

A wide variety of oral and inhaled agents are available for the treatment of asthmatic symptoms. Your physician will work with you to identify those medications that are most suitable for the pattern of disease that you have.

Notify Our Office If

- You develop chronic shortness of breath.
- You note the onset of wheezing when you breathe.
- You have a chronic cough.

Metered-Dose Inhalers

Patient and Caregiver's Guide

General Information

Metered-dose inhalers are commonly used to provide a dose of medication directly into the breathing passages that lead to the lungs. They are often used in patients with asthma, bronchitis, and chronic obstructive pulmonary disease. They must be used properly to get their full effect and to prevent overdosing of the drug administered. The medications administered by metered-dose inhalers are often powerful drugs that must be taken only in the proper dose.

Important Points in Therapy

The inhaler must contain a drug to be effective. Most inhalers are metal canisters, and one cannot see whether they are empty. If you suspect that the inhaler is empty, try floating the canister in a bowl of water. If it sinks, it contains some drug. If it floats, it may be empty. Shake the inhaler well before use. Assemble it according to the manufacturer's instructions.

1. Position the inhaler according to the instructions provided with it. Various kinds of inhalers may require different positions in or in front of the mouth to be effective.
2. Tilt back your head and breathe out as much as possible. Then take a slow, deep breath in, and press the inhaler to release the drug at the same time.
3. Hold the breath in to a count of 10, if possible.
4. Breathe out slowly.
5. If the prescription calls for more than one dose, allow 1 or 2 minutes between doses.
6. Rinse and dry the inhaler and store at room temperature.

Call Our Office If

● You are having difficulty with the use of your inhaler.

Stopping Smoking

Patient and Caregiver's Guide

General Information

Smoking cessation is good preventive health care. It is particularly important for patients suffering from a select list of health problems. This list includes angina pectoris (heart pain), heart attack, chronic obstructive pulmonary disease (including emphysema and/or chronic bronchitis), stroke, dyspepsia, and osteoporosis. You are never too old to gain a benefit from stopping smoking.

Whether you regard smoking as a habit or an addiction, it is a difficult pattern of behavior to stop. There appear to be powerful biochemical urges that induce the chronic smoker to continue to light up. All approaches to smoking cessation must in one way or another address the problem of controlling these urges. What follows is a list of some methods that have worked. They do not all work for everyone. Discuss with your doctor which option might be the most effective for you.

METHODS

Cold turkey	This is the traditional approach. It requires motivation that some people misidentify as will power. Most of the techniques that follow either use some approach to enhance motivation or drugs to mute the urge to smoke.
Tapering off	This involves gradually limiting the number of cigarettes smoked daily. One effective way to do this is to place limits on where you can smoke. Eliminate cigarettes from your car. Do not smoke at the table. Do not smoke at your desk. This is reinforceable if cigarettes are not available at that location. In fact, the fewer cigarettes that you smoke daily the easier it is to stop cold turkey.
Patches	One element of the urge to light up is a falling blood level of nicotine. Nicotine is a drug. It has harmful effects on its own, but these are limited. The tars and other elements of smoke are of

	greater harm than the nicotine. Patches provide a slow release of nicotine through the skin. When the blood level of nicotine does not fall precipitously, it blunts the urge to light up. By slowly changing to patches that provide lower and lower doses of nicotine, this becomes a form of tapering off. Nicotine in patch form is not safe for everyone. Consult your physician concerning the use of this cessation aid.
Gum	Nicotine-containing chewing gum may be used to keep the blood level of nicotine up, which blunts the urge to light up. It permits (and requires) you to control the timing and dose of nicotine. It is another form of tapering off.
Inhalers	A nicotine-containing inhaler, shaped much like a cigarette holder, is available as an additional method to deliver this drug and to help with tapering off.
Drugs	The drug bupropion (Zyban) has been found to be helpful for some people in a program of smoking cessation. How this drug works is not known. It is best used as an adjunct with some form of nicotine replacement. The drug does have side effects and will interact with other medications. It requires a 2- to 3-month course of the drug to be effective. You should consult your physician concerning the safety and possible benefits before attempting to use this drug.
Behavioral modification	Group sessions are a helpful adjunct to any of the stopping smoking program methods. Hypnosis may also be useful for selected individuals.

Notify Our Office If

- You wish to stop smoking or to enter a smoking cessation program.

Pneumonia

Patient and Caregiver's Guide

General Information

Pneumonia is caused by an infection that reaches the tiny air sacs in the lungs, the small passages leading to these air sacs, or both locations. Viruses and fungi cause pneumonia, but most commonly in elderly patients it is caused by bacteria.

Pneumonia may occur at any age, but it is many times (at least five times) more common in elderly patients. In addition, it affects these patients more severely. For generations pneumonia has been a recognized common cause of death in elderly patients. This remains true, despite advances in the treatment of lung infections.

Many different bacteria can infect lung tissue and cause pneumonia. The likely causative organism varies from setting to setting. The infecting bacteria may be inhaled from the air or come from the upper intestinal tract.

Patients with upper respiratory tract infection and influenza viral infection are prone to develop pneumonia. Damaged lungs are more easily infected than healthy lungs. People who smoke and those who are occupationally or environmentally exposed to toxic dust are particularly susceptible. The changes in the aging lungs are enough to increase susceptibility to infection and pneumonia. An additional factor is impaired immunity, particularly in patients receiving steroid medications or cancer chemotherapy, in those with transplanted organs, and in those with acquired immunodeficiency syndrome (AIDS). Any factor, even environmental stress, that may impair resistance leaves the elderly patient vulnerable to pulmonary infection.

Important Points In Treatment

It is best to prevent pneumonia. Vaccines for influenza and for certain pneumococci, organisms that commonly cause pneumonia, are not completely effective but do provide some level of protection.

Careful attention to the treatment of cold and flu is important. Adequate fluids and humidity can help patients bring up secretions and prevent the development of infection in lung tissue. This helps to keep the airways clean and functioning.

Notify Our Office If

- You develop a severe upper respiratory infection or chest cold.
- You cough up blood or yellow phlegm or develop a sudden chest pain.

Influenza Vaccination

Patient and Caregiver's Guide

 ## General Information

Influenza is an annually occurring viral epidemic in the United States and around the world. Most (90%) of the influenza-related deaths occur in the elderly. The primary tool for reducing this death toll is the use of immunization against this virus.

Because the virus changes slightly from year to year, new forms of the virus occur. This means that last year's immunization may not be effective against this year's viruses. Annual immunization is required for it to be effective.

 ## Important Points In Treatment

The annual outbreaks of influenza usually begin in December of each year. The vaccine will require about 2 weeks to become effective. The best time for immunization is in October or November. Protection provided by the vaccine will last about 4 to 6 months. The influenza season in this country ends in March, so one properly timed immunization is usually effective. It requires only a single dose of vaccine.

The site of immunization may be sore for 1 or 2 days after the inoculation. A few patients may have some muscle ache, fever, and tiredness, but this lasts only 1 or 2 days.

The vaccine is made in eggs. Patients who are allergic to eggs or egg products should not take this vaccine.

 ## Notify Our Office If

- You would like to have an immunization against influenza.
- If you seem to have *any kind* of reaction after immunization.

Pneumococcal Immunization

Patient and Caregiver's Guide

General Information

Pneumonia is caused by an infection that reaches the tiny air sacs in the lungs, the small passages leading to these air sacs, or both locations. Viruses and fungi cause pneumonia, but most commonly in elderly patients it is caused by bacteria.

Pneumonia may occur at any age, but it is many times (at least five times) more common in elderly patients. In addition, it affects these patients more severely. For many years, pneumonia has been a recognized common cause of death in elderly patients. This remains true, despite advances in the treatment of lung infections.

Many different bacteria can infect lung tissue and cause pneumonia. The likely causative organism varies from setting to setting. A bacteria called *pneumococcus* is often involved in infections in the elderly.

Vaccination against pneumococcus is effective in preventing much of the pneumonia affecting the elderly. Its use is reported to cause a 70% reduction in this kind of pneumonia in the elderly.

Important Points in Therapy

The pneumococcal vaccine is so potent that it needs to be given only once every 10 years. It requires a single injection. It can be given at the same time as an influenza immunization, but it must be injected at a different site.

The site of immunization may be sore for 1 or 2 days after the inoculation. A few patients may have some muscle ache, fever, and tiredness; but this lasts only 1 or 2 days.

The vaccine is made in eggs. Patients who are allergic to eggs or egg products should not take this vaccine.

Notify Our Office If

- You would like to have a pneumococcal immunization.

Tuberculosis

Patient and Caregiver's Guide

General Information

Tuberculosis is a chronic infection usually involving the lungs but may also involve other organs. About one fourth of newly discovered cases each year occur in elderly patients. Some of these are new infections, but many are recurrences of past infections. New, effective methods of treatment are available and have changed the management of tuberculosis.

For many elderly, the disease is a reactivation of an infection acquired decades before when tuberculosis was a much more common problem. The bacteria remain alive but dormant and can break out to cause new disease when the body's resistance falls. Many other diseases and some treatments of other diseases can cause this impairment of resistance that allows infection to become active. Steroid hormones and anticancer drugs are examples of the kinds of treatments associated with impaired resistance.

The days of prolonged hospitalization in a sanatorium with enforced rest and mutilating operations are gone. An arsenal of new drugs used in outpatient therapy has replaced this older therapy. However, tuberculosis remains a chronic disease, slow in onset and slow to heal, even with the newer drugs. Treatment takes 6 months or longer.

Important Points In Treatment

In the past, sanatorium treatment started with a prolonged period of isolation. This was to prevent the spread of the tubercular bacillus to others by way of bacteria coughed up from the lungs. With the coming of antitubercular drugs, this possible infectious interval is much shorter. Nonetheless, patients with pulmonary tuberculosis should be careful when disposing of paper tissues containing coughed-up secretions. Your physician will advise you when the infectious period is past.

Pulmonary Embolism

Patient and Caregiver's Guide ▮ ▮ ▮

General Information

If a blood clot forms in the circulation in a vein or the heart, it may become dislodged and be carried through the blood vessels, through the heart, and into the lungs. In the lungs, it will become trapped when it plugs a blood vessel. Such a clot formed in the circulation and carried to the lung is a pulmonary embolism.

A pulmonary embolism is dangerous and can lead to death. There is effective treatment, but the problem may be difficult to recognize. No symptom is completely characteristic, but there is a collection of symptoms that, when they occur together, can suggest pulmonary embolism as a diagnosis.

Shortness of breath—a common accompaniment to pulmonary embolism—and chest pain—a particular kind of pain that occurs on taking a deep breath called *pleuritis* or *pleuritic pain*—are common with a pulmonary embolism. Coughing up blood is another significant indicator. Less-specific, but also common, symptoms are fainting, anxiety, unease, and calf pain or swelling, or both.

Important Points In Treatment

The principal treatment is anti-coagulation (blood thinning). Other measures include breathing oxygen to help the heart, relieving anxiety, and relieving pain or discomfort.

Anti-coagulation involves some risk for bleeding. Careful monitoring is needed to ensure that the bleeding tendency is kept inside certain limits. The patient should take anti-coagulant medicines regularly.

Some patients, because of other diseases or problems, are at high risk for bleeding, and other alternatives to anti-coagulation may be considered. Many elderly patients fall into this group.

In some patients it is possible to place a filter in the large vein and carry blood from the legs to the heart. This filter can trap emboli before they reach the lungs. This may be a particularly useful procedure in patients who cannot be considered for anti-coagulation. The filter can be placed with a catheter, and the procedure does not require surgery.

Patients with other diseases that may predispose them to the development of clots and an embolism may require anti-coagulation even though they have not had a pulmonary embolism. This is called *prophylactic anti-coagulation* and is done to prevent clots from forming in a patient at high risk. Patients with atrial fibrillation, venous insufficiency, or a history of thrombophlebitis in the legs are particularly at risk. Patients with a history of one pulmonary embolism are at some risk for a second.

Notify Our Office If

- You develop leg swelling.
- You begin to cough up blood.
- You develop pleuritic chest pain (pain that is made worse or that occurs when you take a breath).

Selective Cough

Patient and Caregiver's Guide

General Information

The cough is the body's way of ridding the upper lung passages and the throat of foreign matter. It helps get rid of secretions and particles as well. Most of us cough in response to a reflex or to a sensation that we have something to expel from our respiratory tree. The changes caused by aging may affect the ability of these mechanisms to work. Coughing becomes less frequent, and problems may occur.

It is wise to cough on purpose, that is, selectively, each morning and evening to help the lungs to remain clean and free of secretions. Patients with chronic lung diseases may need to do selective coughing more frequently to clear their lungs. A selective cough on rising in the morning helps clear any secretions that may have accumulated during sleep. A selective cough before bedtime may help ensure a night of quiet and uninterrupted sleep. A selective cough is a deep-passage clearing cough and is far more effective and less tiring than the chronic cough in response to a tickle in the throat.

Some medications can cause coughing. The drugs used for high blood pressure and other blood vessel problems called *ACE inhibitors* can cause chronic cough. Report chronic cough that is new in onset to your physician.

Important Points In Treatment

- Selective cough is best done seated. Bending forward and leaning on the back of a chair, on a counter, or on a table also makes it easier. Make sure that whatever you lean on is solid and secure so that the cough does not cause you to lose balance or fall.
- When in a comfortable position, take a deep breath in and hold it for just a few seconds. This is not the time to try for a breath-holding record. A few seconds will do perfectly well.

- As an exhalation, cough twice in rapid succession. The first cough starts things out and loosens secretions, and the second cough moves things up and out. Any sputum should be disposed of in a paper tissue.
- If clearance seems incomplete, repeat the selective cough several times. Do not do it so frequently or for so long that it causes you to become tired.

Patients with chronic lung problems, such as bronchitis, may need to lie on one or both sides before coughing to help secretions to drain. This is called *postural drainage*.

Notify Our Office If

- You have a sudden onset of pain in your chest after a cough.
- You notice a sudden onset of shortness of breath after you cough.
- You cough up any blood or tissue.
- You lose consciousness or become dizzy with a cough.

CHAPTER 11

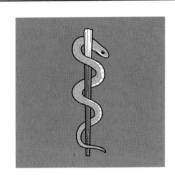
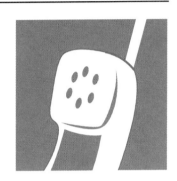

Nutrition

Lactose Intolerance

Patient and Caregiver's Guide

General Information

Lactose is the sugar found in milk. Many people, as they grow older, are unable to digest this sugar because they lose the ability to produce the enzyme lactase in the intestinal tract. This enzyme is essential to permit the digestion of lactose and its absorption into the bloodstream. This problem is called *lactose intolerance*.

When the undigested lactose passes down the intestine into the lower digestive tract, the bacteria normally present in the tract ferments it. This fermentation results in the production of gas and can cause diarrhea.

Many intestinal infections can produce temporary lactase deficiency, but for most people the problem is the permanent reduction in the amount of this enzyme because of aging. The enzyme loss is frequently partial, and the amount remaining varies widely from person to person. Accordingly, the amount of exposure to milk and milk products necessary to produce symptoms varies among individuals.

Important Points in Treatment

Symptoms can be managed in two ways. The first way is to reduce milk and milk products in the diet to levels that are too low to produce symptoms. The severity of the milk-free diet needed varies from person to person with the degree of deficiency of the enzyme lactase. Therefore, trial and error may be necessary to figure out what items to cut from any individual's customary diet. Milk products are hidden in many processed foods, sauces, and breads and other baked goods. Often there are times when avoiding milk products is difficult, if not impossible.

Not all milk products contain lactose in quantities sufficient to produce symptoms. In hard cheeses, such as Swiss or Parmesan, lactose is consumed in the preparation of the cheese, and these products do not produce symptoms. Soft cheeses, such as Brie, may contain more lactose. The fermentation of yogurt also consumes the lactose, converting it into sugars that are readily absorbed in the intestinal tract. Yogurt generally does not produce symptoms of lactose intolerance. Cottage cheese, on the other hand, does contain lactose and can produce symptoms.

The second way to manage lactose intolerance is to add the missing enzyme lactase to milk to predigest the lactose and permit its absorption. This milk may be used for cooking as well as drinking. Also, tablets containing lactase can be taken at the time of eating food that contains milk. This may be helpful when faced with birthday ice cream and cake or a restaurant meal. Many companies are now making lactose-free products, including ice cream.

Caregivers should be aware that traditional nutritional supplements for the ailing individual, including eggnogs, milkshakes, custards, and the like, may contain substantial lactose and may cause symptoms. Lactose content of these preparations is usually listed on the label.

Notify Our Office If

● You have diarrhea that does not resolve.

Cholesterol

Patient and Caregiver's Guide

General Information

Cholesterol and the associated problems that it causes in arterial blood vessels are a concern of adults living in developed countries. It is a preventable and treatable cause of vascular disease. The first changes in the walls of the arteries begin to occur in the teenage years. Many seniors feel that by their fifties, the benefits of preventive treatment are trivial. *This is not true.* Benefits from dietary reduction in cholesterol and other fats accrue in both older and younger patients.

Arteriosclerosis (hardening and narrowing of the arteries), related to elevated cholesterol levels in the blood, progresses if the blood cholesterol remains elevated. This progression can be stopped. Lowering the levels of cholesterol in the blood can slow and at times arrest the further deposition of fat in the walls of the arteries. There is excellent evidence that some of these changes in the walls of the arteries are reversible with stringent dietary management.

Not only does arteriosclerosis narrow the arterial passages, but the fatty deposits may split open or ulcerate, causing a clot to form. A clot of this sort may cause sudden occlusion of the artery. Lowering of the levels of one kind of cholesterol in the blood seems to prevent the development of these splits and ulcers. These are excellent reasons for seniors to be concerned with maintaining a normal blood cholesterol level.

Many patients participate in cholesterol screening programs. These programs use small quantities of blood, often from a simple finger stick, for a rapid test for cholesterol. However, a screening test showing an elevated level is not adequate to permit the diagnosis of elevated blood cholesterol. This is only an indication that a careful test for the various forms of cholesterol in the blood should be done. In patients with borderline levels, several tests may be needed to be sure of the elevation in the cholesterol. Do not undertake treatment with lifestyle modification or powerful drugs, or both, unless the diagnosis of elevated cholesterol is clearly and carefully made.

Cholesterol is a kind of fat. Like all other fats, it mixes poorly with water (or blood). In the blood it attaches to a carrier. There are several kinds of carriers. The simple test for cholesterol measures the total cholesterol in all of the carriers. Your physician may order additional tests to measure the amount of cholesterol associated with each different carrier. The cholesterol associated with one carrier, HDL (high-density lipoprotein), seems to *prevent* the development of arteriosclerosis. The cholesterol associated with two of the carriers, LDL (low-density lipoprotein) and VLDL (very-low-density lipoprotein), seems to be associated with *promoting* the development of arteriosclerosis. Your physician needs to know the kind of cholesterol present to decide whether it is necessary to begin a cholesterol-lowering program.

Important Points in Treatment

The lowering of blood cholesterol can be accomplished by changes in diet and by administration of cholesterol-lowering drugs. Except in patients with very high levels of cholesterol, change in the diet is the preferred initial therapy. Dietary changes cause few, if any, side effects and complications, whereas the drugs used are powerful agents and can cause side effects.

Most adults eat a diet set by custom and lifelong habit. The dietary changes necessary to lower blood cholesterol are major and extensive and require a change in lifelong eating habits. The usual reason for a diet's failure to lower blood cholesterol levels is that it is not *rigorously and carefully followed*. Drug therapy to lower blood cholesterol should always be added to a program of an adequate diet, never substituted for dietary indiscretions.

If you are having problems with your diet, ask your physician for help. Excellent diet books, often with recipes, are available. Books can also be obtained with lists of fat and cholesterol content of prepared and restaurant foods that can help you maintain a diet program at home and when eating out. In selected cases, a discussion with a dietitian may be necessary.

Cholesterol-Lowering Diets

Patient and Caregiver's Guide ▪ ▪ ▪

General Information

Most people eat from a somewhat restricted dietary selection. They eat a traditional, customary, or habitual diet. In the United States, this customary fare has long included large amounts of animal fat in such foods as eggs, milk, butter, pork, and beef. Most people tolerate this diet extremely well. Nonetheless, large numbers of people face the problem of elevated levels of blood cholesterol. Elevated cholesterol levels may cause premature development of hardening of the arteries, atherosclerosis, and the associated problems of heart attack and stroke.

Important Points in Treatment
Dietary Management

The first line of treatment of elevated cholesterol is diet. The dietary changes needed include a long-term change in dietary habits. The change is relatively simple, but because it involves changing a habit, many people find it difficult to accommodate.

Dietary control of blood fats often requires two steps: weight control and change in fat intake. They are equally important and interdependent. The lowering of blood fats works more easily in patients at their ideal weight. Weight reduction is discussed in greater detail in another section (ask for "Weight Loss" and "Obesity and Weight Loss").

Weight reduction results in a fall in blood cholesterol, but this fall is modest at best. Significant changes in blood fat levels require dietary manipulation as well. Careful changes in dietary intake of fats can lower blood fats in all patients, except a few who have inherited high lipid abnormalities. The important information to know concerning your diet is total target calorie intake (to be determined by your physician) and maximum allowed

253

daily fat intake, usually expressed in grams. The goal is to reduce your total daily intake of fat to *30% of your daily calories*, and half the fat should be unsaturated. Knowing your calorie and fat allowance permits you to select a daily menu at home or acceptable restaurant foods.

To be successful, you also need one of the many pocket-sized guides to the calorie and fat content of prepared foods. The handier it is, the greater the likelihood you will have the guide with you when you need it most. Most prepared foods—packaged, frozen, or canned—list nutritional information on the labels. Among items listed are the fat content and the cholesterol content in the food.

Weight Loss

Patient and Caregiver's Guide

General Information

Obesity is common in the United States. A program of weight loss is recommended for many reasons. There is a close relationship between obesity and many diseases. Obesity contributes to the development of hypertension (high blood pressure), wear-and-tear arthritis, and elevated blood cholesterol with its associated problems of hardening of the arteries, heart attacks, and stroke.

Obesity itself is not a disease unless you achieve levels described as *morbid obesity* or *severe obesity.* Probably the best way to evaluate whether or not you are overweight or obese is to use the body mass index, often abbreviated as BMI. It is a calculation based on your weight in kilograms and your height in meters squared. There are many calculators available in both books and on the Internet that permit you to determine your body mass index easily. Individuals who are overweight are defined as having a body mass index between 25 and 29.9. You are classified as obese, if your body mass index is 30 or above. Severe obesity or morbid obesity becomes the diagnosis, if the body mass index is above 40.

The simplicity of the problem of obesity belies the difficulty of its management. Food can be considered the equivalent of fuel. It must be either used or stored after absorption. If you eat more than you need to use, you store the remainder. The storage form is fat. To remain thin, you need to eat no more, on average, than you use, on average. To lose weight, you need to adjust food intake to *less* than the amount of energy you use. The body makes up the difference by withdrawing fat from storage, with a net result of some weight loss.

Almost all nonsurgical weight-loss programs depend on adjusting the dietary intake to include fewer calories. Some programs also address the kinds of foods that you eat and the mix of the various food groups. Some foods are more prone to produce weight gain than others, even if eaten in equal calorie amounts.

Successful weight-loss programs are those that not only result in a loss of weight but also change your eating habits so that you do not regain weight after the diet is finished. One must learn to restrain intake to the amount of food needed to meet daily energy needs and avoid storage as fat.

Weight-loss programs involving surgery utilize a surgical procedure to decrease the size of the stomach and to bypass a portion of the intestine, reducing the absorption of food. If you have severe obesity, particularly with a body mass index over 40, and you have associated diseases or a predisposition to diseases that would be made worse by the obesity, then you may be a candidate for a surgical procedure. This would only be employed if conventional approaches using diet had failed. There is always some risk with surgery, and there are many complications involved in the surgical procedures for obesity. This always requires a risk/benefit analysis.

If you do not have severe obesity or have no associated medical problems, the problem is cosmetic rather than medical. At this point, a risk/benefit analysis is critical.

Important Points in Treatment

Your physician can help you select a regimen of diet and exercise that produces weight loss without being a danger to your health. Several observations may help you adjust to the changes necessary for weight loss.

- Fat deposits accumulate slowly and leave slowly. Day-to-day weight changes are unlikely to be meaningful measures of the effectiveness of your program.
- When fat serves as a source for energy, the chemical reactions that occur produce water. You will not note a loss in weight until the body excretes this water. Some people on a diet may retain water for a week or more before excretion begins and weight loss becomes apparent.
- Recreational exercise alone and exercise for fitness both consume calories, but unless carried to extremes, exercise alone is not an effective weight-control program. Exercise is an effective addition when combined with dietary management for weight control. The levels of exercise appropriate for any individual vary with other health problems and the degree of fitness at the beginning of an exercise program.

Notify Our Office If

- You wish to undertake a weight-loss program.
- You wish to undertake an exercise program.
- You are concerned about possible surgical procedures for weight loss.

Obesity and Weight Loss

Patient and Caregiver's Guide

 ## General Information

Obesity is a frequent feature of the elderly. Some people are overweight throughout their lives, but many more gain weight with the passage of time. A change to a more sedentary lifestyle with retirement is also a factor in weight gain among the elderly. Except for the very svelte, most people will respond to inquiry by indicating they would like to lose some weight. It is no surprise that you can find support for almost any position you wish to take concerning nutrition. Conflicting advice is the rule, not the exception. Although every diet offered for weight loss has demonstrable examples of success, it is also true that no diet is consistently so successful that it has swept the field.

What follows is a common-sense approach to deciding whether you should diet and how you might diet. *Caveat emptor* (let the buyer beware) applies. It is easier to gain weight than it is to lose it.

Should you diet?

Weight loss is only a consideration for the overweight. There are tables that can help you determine whether you are overweight. It is also possible to calculate a figure called the *body mass index* (BMI), which is a good indicator of whether you are overweight.

A second concern is whether there will be a health benefit to weight loss that balances with the personal cost and effort needed to successfully lose weight. There is information indicating that, if you are healthy but overweight when you reach senior years, there may be little benefit to longevity from weight loss. Thus, if you are happy and healthy at your current weight, there may not be a compelling reason to lose weight. There are, however, a number of diseases that are made worse by obesity. There is also the common sense observation that one's quality of life may be enhanced by weight loss. A third observation is that illness—particularly health care emergencies—seems to fall harder on the obese.

Diabetes, hypertension (high blood pressure), hypercholesterolemia (high blood cholesterol), hyperlipidemia (high blood fats), osteoarthritis (wear and tear arthritis), chronic pulmonary disease, heart failure, and a host of other diseases common in the elderly are improved in their management and control by the loss of *excess weight.* The risks imposed by surgery and trauma are less if you are not overweight.

How should you diet?

If you have a medical problem that is, in part or whole, managed by a therapeutic diet, then that is the diet you should follow. Problems with diabetes and high blood fats are the best, but not the only, examples of this form of diet.

If you are dieting primarily for weight loss rather than management of a disease, you will need to select and adopt a diet that you are willing to follow for the rest of your life. Your customary style of eating is what has led you to the obesity that you are trying to reverse. Dieters should understand that once they have successfully lost weight, they will really never be able to return to the pattern of eating that they followed prior to their diet. This does not mean that you must give up forever on a favorite food. It does mean that the frequency with which you can enjoy this particular food will change.

If you adopt a diet that permits you to lose weight but after reaching your target weight you return to your customary diet, you will regain your lost weight. There is little sense, in this case, in trying in the first place. To lose weight, you need to change your customary habit and style of eating, and, to keep the weight off, you must maintain some of this change *forever.* The key to weight-loss success is to select a diet that you can live with. This eliminates most fad diets, diets for which you must buy special foods, or supplements and diets that are relentlessly monotonous.

Five keys to successful dieting

1. Eat when you are hungry, not by the clock or by custom. If your stomach does not tell you it is hungry, don't fill it.
2. Eat slowly. Put your fork down between bites. Don't gorge.
3. Stop when you are full. Don't feel you must clean your plate.
4. Limit your intake of foods that contain sugar or are easily converted to sugar. This includes sweets, sweet drinks,

sweetened desserts, white breads, potatoes, rice, pasta (unless made from whole grain flour), and carrots. Eliminate these to lose weight and limit them to maintain your weight loss.

5. When dieting, some exercise is always beneficial in the weight loss process.

Call Our Office If

- You would like to initiate a weight-loss program.
- You have been given a therapeutic diet but are having difficulty understanding what you should eat and what you should avoid.
- You wish to begin an exercise program.

Trans Fats

Patient and Caregiver's Guide

General Information

Dietary fats are often classified for nutritional purposes as unsaturated fat, saturated fat and trans fat. The amount of each of these kinds of fat that you eat affects the level of cholesterol in your blood in the kind of cholesterol that is circulating. The current suggestion is that fat calories be limited to 30% of your diet. The majority of the fats should be unsaturated fat. Unsaturated fats are largely vegetable fats. Saturated fats, which are commonly associated with animal fats, have deleterious effects on your serum cholesterol levels.

Trans fats may occur naturally in animal fats, but they are also a product of industrial manufacturers of some kinds of shortening and butter substitutes. Although they offer some benefits in cooking, particularly baking, they have a deleterious effect on your serum cholesterol that exceeds that of the ordinary saturated fats.

Many food items now contain on their food label nutritional information that will tell you whether they are high in trans fats. A prudent dieter will avoid these fats whenever possible.

Carbohydrate-Restricted Diets for Weight Loss

Patient and Caregiver's Guide

 ## General Information

The traditional diet program for weight loss involves a diet that is balanced, with fat intake limited to 30% of the calories and with overall calorie restriction. This has been an effective diet for many people, and it is available in many commercial forms that make it easier to diet and follow the various dietary restrictions. Unfortunately, for many people this does not prove to be an effective manner of losing weight.

There are probably a few people who have an unusual metabolism that makes this traditional weight-loss diet less effective, but for most people it is simply not a diet that they are comfortable following. If the traditional program is not effective for you, there are some options. One of these options is a carbohydrate-restricted diet. This form of dieting for weight loss has been used for almost 150 years. It has recent popularity, which has caused many individuals to think of it as a fad diet. Indeed, on the market there are some carbohydrate-restricted diets that involve very specific restrictions. These would properly be called *fad diets.*

A simple carbohydrate–restricted diet can be very effective in the control of weight. Many individuals who are not comfortable with the traditional weight-loss diet find the carbohydrate-restricted diet much easier to follow. This diet is based on the information that large amounts of carbohydrate quickly converted into easily absorbed sugar in your intestine resulted in a deposition of fat rather than total consumption of all of the calories by your metabolism. Restricting carbohydrate intake avoids this fat deposition.

The usual approach to identifying foods that are high in absorbable carbohydrate is the use of the glycemic index. This is a nutritional tool that assigns a number to each kind of food. The higher the number, the more likely it is that the food contains substantial absorbable carbohydrate. A simple carbohydrate-restricted diet would use the glycemic index to select foods with a low value and avoid foods with a high value.

In addition to this it is important to remember that one still needs to restrict the total number of calories in each day. This is easily done by limiting yourself to a single helping in three regular meals a day.

Many of the commercial carbohydrate-restricted diets begin with an induction period that involves severe carbohydrate restriction and promotes a rapid start to the weight loss. This is probably not essential for the carbohydrate-restricted diet to be effective. What *is* essential is that, to lose weight, you must restrict your ingestion of carbohydrates that are absorbable to a level that induces weight loss. Then you must continue this diet until you have reached your target weight. Once you reach that weight you may cautiously add back carbohydrates until you reach the point where weight loss stops. You then have a dietary level of carbohydrate that you must follow to prevent regaining the weight.

This does not mean that you never get to eat a favorite carbohydrate-containing food again. You can but you must compensate in the following days by additional carbohydrate restriction to restore your ideal weight. There is no question that *you will never be able to return to the pattern of eating that you followed prior to your dietary weight loss.* Once you become familiar with the glycemic index, such compensation becomes almost automatic. This permits you to enjoy family and holiday events without destroying your weight maintenance program. A brief glycemic index follows. More complete and more elaborate listings can be found on the Internet or in many publications.

Foods are listed from highest to lowest glycemic index within each category. Glycemic index was calculated using glucose as the reference with glycemic index of 100. (The University of Sidney, www.glycemicindex.com)
No endorsement of companies or their products is intended and criticism is not implied of similar companies or their products that are not included.

Breads & Grains
Waffle—76
Doughnut—76
Bread, whole wheat—73
Bagel—72
Wheat bread, white—70
Cornmeal —68
Bran muffin—60
Rice, white—56
Rice, brown—55
Wheat kernels—48
Rice, instant (1 minute)—46
Bulgur—46
Spaghetti, white—41
Spaghetti, whole wheat—32
Barley—25

Cereals
Rice Krispies—82
Grape Nuts Flakes—80
Cornflakes—77
Cheerios—74
Shredded Wheat—67
Grape Nuts—67
Life—66
All Bran—38

Fruits
Watermelon—72
Pineapple—66
Raisins—64
Banana—51
Orange—48
Grapes—43
Apple—40
Pear—33

Starchy Vegetables
Carrots—92
Potatoes, instant—88
Potatoes, baked—78
Potatoes, mashed—73
Sweet potatoes—48

Legumes
Baked beans—40
Butter beans—36
Split peas—32
Lentils—28
Kidney beans—23
Soy beans—15

Dairy
Ice cream—62
Yogurt, low fat sweetened—33

Milk, skim—32
Milk, full fat—2

Snacks
Rice cakes—82
Jelly beans—80
Graham crackers—74
Life Savers—70
Angel food cake—67
Wheat crackers—67
Potato chips—57
Popcorn—55
Oatmeal cookies—54
Banana cake—47
Chocolate—44
Corn chips—42
Peanuts—13

Sugars
Honey—87
Sucrose—60
Lactose—43
Fructose—20

Beverages
Soft drinks—63
Orange juice—57
Apple juice—41

For additional glycemic indexes, visit these Web sites:
www.diabetesdigest.com/dd_nutrition2.htm
www.diabetesnet.com/diabetes_food_diet/glycemic_index.php
www.mesquitemagic.com/glycemic_Index_chart.htm

Prepared by Karin Westberg, graduate student; Ruth Litchfield, Ph.D., R.D., extension nutritionist; and Diane Nelson, extension communication specialist. Iowa State University of Science and Technology, Ames, Iowa.

Malnutrition

Patient and Caregiver's Guide ▪ ▪ ▪

General Information

Even in an environment in which there is ample food available to eat, older patients may still experience malnutrition. Such malnutrition may represent a failure to eat or may involve a deficiency in a specific element, such as a single vitamin. As with most health problems, it is better to prevent malnutrition than to treat it. Each of us has food likes and dislikes. For the older patient, it is a short step from picky eating to poor nutrition. The common causes of poor nutrition are given below. Correction begins with recognizing the potential causes. Often several factors, none alone serious enough to be a problem, combine to produce true malnutrition.

Aging factors

Activity often decreases with advancing age. Appetite seems to wane with the decrease in exercise. It is common for older patients to lose weight. In addition, changes in the teeth, particularly poorly fitting dentures, may make eating uncomfortable, subtly leading to decreased total food intake.

Age-related changes in the digestive tract, particularly in the swallowing mechanism, can cause avoidance of some foods. Grilled meats and soft white bread are particularly hard to swallow. Combinations of difficulty with chewing and swallowing may result in a diet so restricted in variety that specific vitamin or mineral deficiencies develop.

Environmental factors

Aging produces major environmental changes. Isolation because of loss of mobility, loss of spouse, or depression impairs the willingness to prepare food and to eat regularly and well. The loss of social contacts alone can be enough to impair nutrition. The substitution of institutional food may not resolve the problem. In

---

fact, bland foods and the loss of traditional favorites may worsen intake. Poverty is an ever-present issue affecting the ability to obtain and prepare an adequate diet.

Disease factors

Disease affects nutritional needs both directly and indirectly. Almost any disease process increases the body's energy needs. Most younger people meet this need by increasing their food intake. Older patients may be too debilitated to respond. In addition, as mentioned previously, they may lack the appetite response. Serious illness is a nutritional burden.

Illnesses that involve the digestive tract may directly impair the ability to eat. These diseases may impair the ability to digest and absorb food as well. These problems in nutrition are the most severe, but they are also usually the most apparent.

Some medications can interfere with appetite. Also, some foods may interfere with the absorption of medications. The timing of meals and medications can be important to treatment. Many patients are placed on a restrictive diet to help in their treatment. The worst problems occur with the imposition of several restrictions at once. A patient placed on a pureed, low-fat, low-salt diet has very restricted food choices. Often only the help of a professional dietitian can sort out these choices into tasty, acceptable food.

Important Points in Treatment

For the caregiver: Visit patients while they are eating on a frequent, but not necessarily regular, basis. The feature to look for is whether they have changed their customary eating habits. If they are not eating what they used to eat, they are probably not eating as much as they used to eat. The correct intervention is not always easy to determine. The following checklist may help:

- Is help needed for shopping?
- Is help needed for menu selection?
- Is help needed for food preparation?
- Is help needed for the act of eating?
- Does the patient need company during meals?
- Will a dietitian help?
- Is a visit to the physician necessary?

Diets

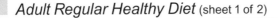

PURPOSE

This diet is designed to promote optimum health through good nutrition. It is to be used for those individuals requiring no special dietary modification or restrictions.

DESCRIPTION

Foods from all basic food groups are included with the addition of other foods to meet energy needs and provide essential nutrients. The diet is planned to promote the prevention of chronic diseases, such as heart disease, cancer, and diabetes.

BASIC INFORMATION

The Dietary Guidelines for Americans outlines what people should eat to stay healthy. The guidelines include:

- eating a variety of foods.
- maintaining a healthy weight.
- choosing a diet low in fat, saturated fat, and cholesterol.
- using sugars only in moderation.
- choosing a diet with plenty of vegetables, fruits, and grain products.
- using salt and sodium in moderation only.
- drinking alcoholic beverages in moderation only.

The United States Department of Agriculture (USDA) Food Guide Pyramid is a diet plan to help individuals meet the dietary guidelines. Each of these food groups provides some, but not all, of the nutrients that people need. Foods in one group cannot replace those in another. For good health all are needed.

The Food Guide Pyramid emphasizes foods from these food groups:

- Bread, cereal, rice, and pasta (6–11 servings daily)
All of these foods are from grains. Individuals need the most of these foods each day.

- Vegetables (3–5 servings daily) & fruits (2–4 servings daily)
All of these foods are from plants. Most people need to eat more of these foods for the vitamins, minerals, and fiber they supply. Examples of a serving are 1 orange, ½ cup juice, ½ medium cantaloupe, ½ cup vegetables or fruit. Good sources of vitamin A (beta carotene) are dark green or dark yellow vegetables. Good sources of vitamin C are citrus fruits, tomatoes, peppers, potatoes, and various greens.

- Milk, yogurt, cheese (2–3 servings daily) & meat, poultry, fish, dry beans, eggs, nuts (2–3 servings daily)
Most of these foods come from animals. These foods are important for protein, calcium, iron, and zinc.

- Fats, oils, & sweets (use sparingly)
These foods provide calories and little else nutritionally. Most people should use these foods sparingly.

NUTRITIONAL ADEQUACY

This diet is designed to provide adequate amounts of calories, vitamins, minerals, and other nutrients to meet the nutritional needs of healthy adults.

Suggested Meal Plan	Suggested Foods and Beverages
Breakfast Fruit Juice Cereal Meat/Meat Substitute Bread/Margarine Milk Beverage	 Orange Juice Oatmeal Scrambled Eggs Whole Wheat Toast/Jelly/Margarine* Skim Milk Coffee or Tea
Dinner—Noon or Evening Meal Meat Substitute Potato/Potato Substitute Vegetable and/or Salad Bread/Margarine Dessert Beverage	 Baked Chicken Sweet Potatoes Green Beans, Coleslaw Whole Wheat Bread, Margarine* Strawberries Coffee or Tea
Supper—Evening or Noon Meal Soup or Juice Meat/Meat Substitute Potato/Potato Substitute Vegetable and/or Salad Bread/Margarine Dessert Milk/Beverage	 Vegetable/Bean Soup Meatballs with Tomato Sauce Spaghetti Broccoli, Spinach Salad/Dressing* Garlic Bread Rice Pudding Skim Milk

*To reduce the fat in your diet, omit margarine and use nonfat salad dressing.

Nutrient Analysis

Calories	2271 Kcal	Riboflavin	2.4 mg
Protein	109 gm	Thiamin	1.7 mg
Carbohydrate	299 gm	Folate	381 mcg
Fat	77 gm	Calcium	1283 mg
Cholesterol	386 mg	Phosphorus	1931 mg
Dietary Fiber	31 gm	Zinc	7 mg
Vitamin A	4570 RE	Iron	18 mg
Vitamin C	249 mg	Sodium	3784 mg
Niacin	25 mg	Potassium	4580 mg

From Griffith HW. Instructions for Patients, 5th ed. Philadelphia, WB Saunders, 1994, pp 506–507. Adapted from Arizona Diet Manual (revised 1992).

A well-balanced diet is as essential in this age group as it is in any other. Because metabolism is decreased in older people, you probably will not require as many calories per day as do younger people. We suggest that you eat small meals every 5 hours or so. Do not let more than 14 hours pass between having a substantial evening meal and breakfast.

We recommend 2400 calories per day for men of normal weight, capable of normal activity, who are 51 years of age or older. For women in this same age group, 1800 calories should be ample.

Sample General Diet

Suggested Meal Plan	Sample Menu
Breakfast	
Citrus fruit or juice	Orange juice
Cereal	Oatmeal
Meat or meat substitute	Soft-cooked eggs
Bread—butter or margarine	Toast—butter or margarine—jelly
Milk	Milk
Beverage	Coffee or tea
Dinner (Noon or Evening Meal)	
Meat or meat substitute	Baked meat loaf with gravy
Potato or potato substitute	Whipped potatoes
Vegetable and/or	Buttered green beans
salad	Tossed green salad with oil and vinegar dressing
Dessert	Lemon sponge pudding
Bread—butter or margarine	Bread—butter or margarine
Beverage	Coffee or tea
Supper (Evening or Noon Meal)	
Soup or juice	Consommé
Meat or meat substitute	Creamed chicken on toast
Vegetable and/or	Buttered peas
salad	Sliced tomato on lettuce leaf with mayonnaise
Dessert	Baked apple with cinnamon
Bread—butter or margarine	Bread—butter or margarine
Milk	Milk
Beverage	Coffee or tea

From Griffith HW. Instructions for Patients, 4th ed. Philadelphia, WB Saunders, 1989, p 91. Adapted from Arizona Diet Manual (4th ed, 1985).

PURPOSE

The low-cholesterol, low-sodium diets are designed to help reduce serum lipids and to achieve a reduction in sodium intake that may be necessary for the control of hypertension or other disorders.

DESCRIPTION

This diet meets the general requirements of the National Cholesterol Education Program. Foods high in total fat, saturated fat, and cholesterol are controlled. Total cholesterol intake is restricted. Limited amounts of monounsaturated and polyunsaturated fats are used as replacements for saturated fats. Calories need to be adjusted to achieve or maintain desired body weight.

Foods high in sodium content are omitted. One-half teaspoon of salt is allowed in the preparation of food or may be used at the table. As the quantities of allowed foods are not restricted, the level of sodium may vary.

BASIC INFORMATION

Cholesterol is found in animal products only. Saturated fats are often solid at room temperature and are usually found in animal products, such as meats, poultry, butter, cheese, and ice cream. Plant sources of saturated fats include palm oil, palm kernel oil, and coconut oil. Monounsaturated fats are found in products, such as olive oil, peanuts, flaxseed oil, and canola (rapeseed) oil. Polyunsaturated fats are usually liquid at room temperature and are found in safflower, sunflower, corn, soybean, and cottonseed oils.

Salt-free herbs and spices may be used freely. Carefully read labels because some salt-replacement seasonings contain sodium chloride. "Light" salts, which are a mixture of potassium chloride and sodium chloride, are also limited on sodium-controlled diets.

NUTRITIONAL ADEQUACY

Depending on an individual's food choices, the low-cholesterol, low-sodium diets will normally be adequate in all nutrients.

FOOD LISTS

Milk/Dairy (limit to 2–3 servings a day)
• **Allowed:** Skim (nonfat) or 1% fat milk (liquid, powdered, evaporated); nonfat or low-fat yogurt, low-fat cottage cheese (2% fat or less), low-fat cheese (labeled 6 grams of fat or less per ounce); nonfat sour cream.
• **Avoid:** Whole milk (4% fat) (liquid, evaporated, condensed); 2% milk, cream, half-and-half, imitation milk products, most nondairy creamers, whipped toppings; whole milk yogurt; regular cottage chesse (4% fat); natural cheeses made from whole milk (cheddar, Swiss, blue, Camembert, etc.); cream cheese; sour cream; low fat cream cheese; low fat sour cream. NOTE: If 2% milk is used, decrease added fat by 1 teaspoon for each cup of milk.

Meat/Meat Substitute (limit to 5 oz. a day from animal products; limit four egg yolks a week)
• **Allowed:** Dried beans, split peas, lentils, pinto beans cooked without salt; poultry without the skin; fish; tuna packed in water; lean beef (extra lean ground beef, eye of round, sirloin, round tip, round, top round, tenderloin, top loin); lean pork (fresh not cured, tenderloin, leg, shoulder); lamb (arm, leg, loin, rib); shrimp or lobster (limit 3 oz. per week); luncheon meats (1 gram fat or less per ounce); egg whites (two egg whites = one whole egg); low cholesterol egg substitutes.
• **Avoid:** Fried meats or meat substitutes; any meat, fish, or poultry that is smoked, cured, salted, or canned (e.g., bacon, dried beef, corned beef, cold cuts, ham, turkey ham, hot dogs, sausages, sardines, anchovies, pickled herring); fatty cuts of beef, pork, lamb; goose, duck; liver, kidney, brains, or other organ meats; sausage, bacon; regular luncheon meats; egg yolks.

Breads & Grains (6–11 servings a day)
• **Allowed:** Whole-grain breads (oatmeal, whole wheat, rye, bran, multigrain, etc.); rice, pasta; homemade baked goods low in fat; low-fat crackers (rice cakes, popcorn cakes, Ry Krisp, melba toast, pretzels, breadsticks); hot or cold cereals (with no fat).
• **Avoid:** High-fat baked goods (pies, cakes, doughnuts, croissants, pastries, muffins, biscuits); high-fat crackers; egg noodles; granola-type cereals; cereals with more than 2 grams of fat per serving; pasta and rice prepared with cream, butter, or cheese sauces; breads, rolls, and crackers with salted tops; instant rice and pasta mixes; commercial stuffing; commercial casserole mixes.

FOOD LISTS (continued)

Vegetables (3–5 servings or more per day)
• **Allowed:** Any fresh, frozen, dried, or low-sodium (canned); regular canned, drained vegetables—limit to 1 serving per day; low-salt vegetable juices.
• **Avoid:** Vegetables prepared in butter, cream, or other sauces; fried vegetables; sauerkraut; pickled vegetables and others prepared in brine; regular vegetable juice; potato casserole mixes; regular and salt-free potato chips.

Fruits (4 servings or more per day)
• **Allowed:** Any fresh, frozen, canned, or dried.
• **Avoid:** Coconuts, avocados, and olives, except as allowed under "miscellaneous."

Desserts & Sweets (Limit to control calories)
• **Allowed:** Sugar, jelly, jam, honey, molasses; low-fat frozen desserts (e.g., sherbet, sorbet, ices, nonfat frozen yogurt, popsicles); angel food cake; low-fat cakes and cookies (e.g., vanilla wafers, graham crackers, ginger snaps); baking cocoa; low-fat candy (e.g., jelly beans, hard candy).
• **Avoid:** Ice cream; high-fat cakes, pies, and cookies (most commercially made); chocolate.

Beverages
• **Allowed:** Juices, tea, coffee, decaffeinated coffee, carbonated drinks, most alcoholic beverages.
• **Avoid:** Milkshakes; ice cream floats; eggnog; alcoholic beverages containing milk, cream or coconut; commercially softened water as beverage or in food preparation.

Miscellaneous
• **Allowed:** Limit fat based on total number of calories consumed (use very sparingly). Limit (1 tsp per serving): Unsaturated vegetable oils (corn, olive, canola, safflower, sesame, soybean, sunflower); margarine or shortening made from unsaturated vegetable oils; mayonnaise and salad dressings made from unsaturated oils (1 Tbsp); diet margarine (1 tsp), salt-free seeds and nuts (1 Tbsp seeds, 6 almonds, 20 small peanuts).

No Limit: Vegetable oil sprays; fat-free salad dressings; herbs, spices, pepper, salt substitute with physician approval; mustard; vinegar; lemon and lime juice; cream sauces made with allowed ingredients.

Limit added salt to ½ teaspoon per day; may be used in cooking or at the table.
• **Avoid:** Butter; coconut oil; palm oil; palm kernel oil; lard; bacon fat; salad dressings made with egg yolk; fried snack foods (potato chips, cheese curls, tortilla chips); olives; avocados; regular cream sauces; salt, garlic salt, celery salt, onion salt, seasoned salt, sea salt, kosher salt; seasonings containing monosodium glutamate (MSG, Accent); salted nuts and seeds; salted peanut butter, canned soups.

SAMPLE MENU

Suggested Meal Plan	Suggested Foods and Beverages
Breakfast Fruit Juice Cereal Meat/Meat Substitute Bread/Margarine Milk Beverage	Grapefruit Half Bran Flakes Low Cholesterol Egg Substitute 2 Slices Whole Wheat Toast 1 tsp Margarine/Jelly 1 cup 1% Milk Coffee
Dinner—Noon or Evening Meal Meat/Meat Substitute Potato/Potato Substitute Vegetable and/or Salad Bread/Margarine Dessert Beverage	3 oz. Salt-Free, Fat-Free Chicken Breast Salt-Free, Fat-Free Sweet Potato Salt-Free, Fat-Free Green Beans Whole Wheat Bread/Margarine Strawberries Iced Tea

Supper—Evening or Noon Meal
Soup or Juice
Meat/Meat Substitute
 	
Potato Substitute
Vegetable and/or
  Salad
Bread/Margarine
Dessert
Milk
Beverage
	½ cup Salt-Free Vegetable Juice
	3 oz. Salt-Free, Fat-Free Meatballs in Salt-Free
	  Tomato Sauce
	Spaghetti
	Salt-Free, Fat-Free Broccoli, Spinach Salad, 1 Tbsp
	  Dressing
	Garlic Bread, 1 tsp Margarine
	Fruit Sorbet
	1 cup 1% Milk
	Coffee or Tea

Other: Can use up to ½ teaspoon salt in cooking or at the table.

Nutrient Analysis

Calories	1815 Kcal	Riboflavin	2.9 mg
Protein	96 gm	Thiamin	1.8 mg
Carbohydrate	240 gm	Folate	529 mcg
Fat	58 gm	Calcium	999 mg
Cholesterol	171 mg	Phosphorus	1541 mg
Dietary Fiber	39 gm	Zinc	13 mg
Vitamin A	4699 RE	Iron	21 mg
Vitamin C	285 mg	Sodium	2936 mg
Niacin	33 mg	Potassium	3507 mg

From Griffith HW. Instructions for Patients, 5th ed. Philadelphia, WB Saunders, 1994, pp 515–517. Adapted from Arizona Diet Manual (revised 1992).

PURPOSE

The low-fat, low-cholesterol diets are designed to reduce serum lipids for the treatment and prevention of coronary heart disease (CHD). It is believed, and recent studies support the idea, that lowering the levels of cholesterol in the blood will prevent the formation of fatty plaques found in the thickening of the artery walls, known as *atherosclerosis*.

DESCRIPTION

Foods high in total fat, saturated fat, and cholesterol are controlled. Total cholesterol intake is restricted. Limited amounts of monounsaturated and polyunsaturated fats are used as replacements for saturated fats. Calories need to be adjusted to achieve or maintain desired body weight. Lean meat, fish, skinless poultry, non- or low-fat dairy products are included. Fatty meat, organ meats, egg yolks, and cheese are limited. Foods high in complex carbohydrates and fiber, such as fruits, vegetables, whole grain products, and legumes are emphasized.

BASIC INFORMATION

The National Cholesterol Education Program (NCEP) Guidelines indicate that a serum total cholesterol should be measured in all adults over the age of 20 at least once every 5 years. Levels below 100 mg/dl are classified as "desirable blood cholesterol," those 130 to 159 mg/dl as "borderline high cholesterol" and those 160 mg/dl as "high blood cholesterol."

Dietary treatment is the primary treatment for elevated serum cholesterol. The goals of therapy are to reduce serum cholesterol to less than 130 mg/dl and low density lipoprotein (LDL) to less than 100 mg/dl. Another goal of therapy is to maintain a nutritionally adequate eating pattern.

Diet Therapy of Blood Cholesterol

Nutrient	Recommended Intake
Total fat	Less than 30% of total calories
Saturated fat	Less than 10% of total calories
Polyunsaturated fat	Up to 10% of total calories
Monounsaturated fat	10%–15% of total calories
Carbohydrates	50%–60% of total calories
Protein	10%–20% of total calories
Cholesterol	Less than 300 mg
Total calories	To achieve and maintain desirable weight

Cholesterol is found in animal products only. Saturated fats are often solid at room temperature and are usually found in animal products, such as meats, poultry, butter, cheese, and ice cream. Plant sources of saturated fats include palm oil, palm kernel oil, and coconut oil. Monounsaturated fats are found in products, such as olive oil, peanuts, flaxseed oil, and canola (rapeseed) oil. Polyunsaturated fats are usually liquid at room temperature and are found in safflower, sunflower, corn, soybean, and cottonseed oils.

Along with cholesterol testing, all adults should be evaluated for other CHD risk factors, such as hypertension, smoking, diabetes, obesity, and family history.

FOOD LISTS

Milk/Dairy (limit to 2–4 servings a day)
• **Allowed:** Skim (nonfat) or 1% fat milk (liquid, powdered, evaporated); nonfat or low-fat yogurt, low-fat cottage cheese (2% fat or less), low-fat cheese (labeled 6 grams of fat or less per ounce); nonfat sour cream; nonfat cream cheese.
• **Avoid:** Whole milk (4% fat) (liquid, evaporated, condensed), 2% milk, cream, half-and-half, imitation milk products, most nondairy creamers, whipped toppings; whole milk yogurt; regular cottage cheese (4% fat); natural cheeses made from whole milk (cheddar, Swiss, blue, Camembert, etc); cream cheese; goat's milk cheese; sour cream; low-fat cream cheese; low-fat sour cream. NOTE: If 2% milk is used, decrease added fat by 1 teaspoon for each cup of milk.

FOOD LISTS (continued)

Meat/Meat Substitute (limit to 5 oz. a day from animal products; limit four egg yolks a week)
• **Allowed:** Dried beans, split peas, lentils, pinto beans cooked without salt; poultry without the skin; fish; tuna packed in water; lean beef (extra lean ground beef, eye of round sirloin, round tip, round, top round, tenderloin, top loin); lean pork (fresh not cured, tenderloin, leg, shoulder); lamb (arm, leg, loin, rib); shrimp or lobster (limit 3 oz. per week); luncheon meats (1 gram fat or less per ounce); egg whites (two egg whites = one whole egg); low cholesterol egg substitutes.
• **Avoid:** Fried meats or meat substitutes; fatty cuts of beef, pork, lamb, goose, duck; liver, kidney, brains, or other organ meats; hot dogs, sausages, bacon; regular luncheon meats; peanut butter; egg yolks.

Breads & Grains (6–11 servings a day)
• **Allowed:** Whole-grain breads (oatmeal, whole wheat, rye, bran, multigrain, etc.); rice, pasta; homemade baked goods low in fat; low-fat crackers (rice cakes, popcorn cakes, Ry Krisp, melba toast, pretzels, breadsticks); hot or cold cereals (with 1 to 2 grams of fat or less per serving).
• **Avoid:** High-fat baked goods (pies, cakes, doughnuts, croissants, pastries, muffins, biscuits); high-fat crackers; egg noodles; granola-type cereals; cereals with more than 2 grams of fat per serving; pasta and rice prepared with cream, butter, or cheese sauces.

Vegetables (3–5 servings or more per day)
• **Allowed:** Any fresh, frozen, canned or dried.
• **Avoid:** Vegetables prepared in butter, cream or other sauces; fried vegetables.

Fruits (4 servings or more per day)
• **Allowed:** Any fresh, frozen, canned, or dried.
• **Avoid:** Coconuts, avocados, and olives, except as allowed under "miscellaneous."

Desserts & Sweets (limit to control calories)
• **Allowed:** Sugar, jelly, jam, honey, molasses; low-fat frozen desserts (e.g., sherbet, sorbet, ices, nonfat frozen yogurt, popsicles); angel food cake; low-fat cakes and cookies (e.g., vanilla wafers, graham crackers, ginger snaps); baking cocoa; low-fat candy (e.g., jelly beans, hard candy).
• **Avoid:** Ice cream; high-fat cakes, pies, and cookies (most commercially made); chocolate.

Beverages
• **Allowed:** Juices, tea, coffee, decaffeinated coffee, carbonated drinks, most alcoholic beverages.
• **Avoid:** Milkshakes; ice cream floats; eggnog; alcoholic beverages containing milk, cream or coconut; commercially softened water as beverage or in food preparation.

Miscellaneous
• **Allowed:** Limit fat based on total number of calories consumed. Generally no more than 6–8 servings/day of added fat, such as margarine and salad dressings, should be eaten; overweight, sedentary, or elderly individuals may need less.
  Limit: (1 tsp per serving) Unsaturated vegetable oils (e.g., corn, canola, flaxseed, safflower, sesame, soybean, sunflower); margarine or shortening made from unsaturated vegetable oils; mayonnaise and salad dressings made from unsaturated oils (1 Tbsp); diet margarine (2 tsp); avocado (⅛ medium or 2 Tbsp); salt-free seeds and nuts (1 Tbsp seeds, 6 almonds, 20 small peanuts); salt-free peanut butter (2 tsp).
  No Limit: Vegetable oil sprays; fat-free salad dressings; herbs, spices, pepper, salt substitute with physician approval; mustard; vinegar; lemon and lime juice; cream sauces made with allowed ingredients.
• **Avoid:** Butter; coconut oil; palm oil; palm kernel oil; lard; bacon fat; salad dressings made with egg yolk; fried snack foods (e.g., potato chips, cheese curls, tortilla chips); olives; avocados; regular cream sauces.

FOOD LISTS (continued)

SAMPLE MENU

Suggested Meal Plan	Suggested Foods and Beverages
Breakfast Fruit Juice Cereal Meat/Meat Substitute Bread/Margarine Milk Beverage	Grapefruit Half Bran Flakes Low-Cholesterol Egg Substitute 2 Slices Whole Wheat Toast, 1 tsp Jelly 1 cup 1% Milk[*] Coffee
Dinner—Noon or Evening meal Meat/Meat Substitute Potato/Potato Substitute Vegetable and/or Salad Bread/Margarine Dessert Beverage	3 oz. Fat-Free Chicken Breast Fat-Free Sweet Potato Fat-Free Green Beans Whole Wheat Bread, Margarine[*] Strawberries Iced Tea
Supper—Evening or Noon Meal Soup or Juice Meat/Meat Substitute Potato Substitute Vegetable and/or Salad Bread/Margarine Dessert Milk Beverage	½ cup Salt-Free Vegetable Juice 3 oz. Fat-Free Meatballs in Tomato Sauce Spaghetti Fat-Free Broccoli Garlic Bread, 1 tsp Margarine[*] Fruit Sorbet 1 cup 1% Milk[*] Coffee or Tea

[*]To further reduce amount of fat in your diet, omit margarine and use skim milk.

Nutrient Analysis

Calories	1781 Kcal	Riboflavin	2.8 mg
Protein	97 gm	Thiamin	2.5 mg
Carbohydrate	255 gm	Folate	589 mcg
Fat	62 gm	Calcium	888 mg
Cholesterol	132 mg	Phosphorus	2111 mg
Dietary Fiber	42 gm	Zinc	20 mg
Vitamin A	2885 RE	Iron	23 mg
Vitamin C	248 mg	Sodium	2803 mg
Niacin	39 mg	Potassium	4579 mg

From Griffith HW. Instructions for Patients, 5th ed. Philadelphia, WB Saunders, 1994, pp 519–521. Adapted from Arizona Diet Manual (revised 1992).

PURPOSE

Sodium-controlled diets are used to reduce blood pressure in hypertension and to promote the loss of excess fluids in edema due to cardiovascular or renal disease and in ascites due to hepatic disease. Sodium-controlled diets may also enhance the action of some medications.

DESCRIPTION 2.0–2.5 grams sodium (86–109 mEq Na)

This level of sodium is used for low-salt, low-sodium, salt-free, and no-salt diet prescriptions. Foods high in sodium content are omitted. One-fourth teaspoon of salt is allowed in the preparation of food or may be used at the table. Since sodium is widely distributed in foods, portions and number of servings are restricted according to the sodium content.

BASIC INFORMATION

Salt substitutes should be approved by the physician. Salt-free herbs and spices may be used freely. Carefully reading labels is important because some salt-replacement seasonings contain sodium chloride. "Light" salts that are a mixture of potassium chloride and sodium chloride are also limited on sodium-controlled diets.

Approximately 75% of the sodium Americans consume is added to foods during processing. The following list will help you interpret sodium information on food labels:
- Sodium-free—5 mg or less of sodium per serving
- Very low sodium—35 mg or less of sodium per serving
- Low sodium—140 mg or less of sodium per serving
- Reduced sodium—75% less sodium than the original version of the product
- No added salt or unsalted—no salt is added during processing (but this does not guarantee that the food product is naturally low in sodium)

Water Supply

Water supplies vary in natural sodium content. For the sodium content in your water supply, call your city's Water Department. Water softeners may add large amounts of sodium to the water. The sodium content of softened water ranges between 7 and 220 milligrams per quart. The company that installed your softener can tell you how much sodium is in your system. Distilled drinking water may be used for cooking and drinking when water supplies more than 120 mg sodium per liter and the diet is below 2.5 grams.

Recommended Intake

The estimated average daily intake of sodium in the American diet ranges from 4 to 5.8 grams per day. The American Heart Association recommends that sodium intake should not exceed 3 grams per day. The National Heart, Lung and Blood Institute recommends a maximum of 3.3 grams of sodium for healthy adults.

Hypertension (High Blood Pressure)

Treatment for hypertension is not limited to taking medicines and the control of sodium intake. Lifestyle and dietary treatments also play a role:
- Cigarette smoking cessation
- Weight reduction (if overweight)
- Excessive alcohol intake reduction
- Stress reduction
- Increased aerobic exercise
- Generous intakes of potassium and calcium
- Correction of magnesium deficiency

Although the medical management of high blood pressure has greatly improved, not all clients are benefited by and/or can tolerate antihypertensive drugs. Changing lifestyle or diet will often result in a reduction in drug requirements and thereby decrease costs and adverse reactions.

Approximately 10% of the population has elevated blood pressure that is markedly affected by salt. Scientific debate continues about recommendations for everyone to cut back on salt. There is still a great deal to be learned about how salt impacts on blood pressure. There is no simple inexpensive test to learn who is salt sensitive. Most experts believe it would be prudent to limit sodium intake. It is especially important for many elderly Americans, African Americans, and those already afflicted with hypertension. American Indians, especially those who develop the nephropathy of diabetes mellitus, are also at particular risk of high blood pressure.

FOOD LISTS

Milk/Dairy (1–4 servings/day)
- **Allowed:** Any milk—white, low-fat, skim, chocolate and cocoa; yogurt; eggnog, ice cream, sherbet, natural cheese (limit 1 oz. per day). Substitute for 8 oz. of milk: 4 oz. evaporated milk, 4 oz. condensed milk, ⅓ cup dry milk powder.
- **Avoid:** Buttermilk, malted milk.

Meats/Meat Substitute (6 oz./day)
- **Allowed:** Fresh or fresh frozen: beef, lamb, pork, veal, and game: chicken, turkey, Cornish hen, or other poultry; any fresh-water or fresh-frozen unbreaded fish and shellfish; low-sodium canned tuna or salmon; low-sodium peanut butter; eggs, dried beans, and peas.
- **Avoid:** Any meat, fish, or poultry that is smoked, cured, salted, or canned, such as bacon, dried beef, corned beef, cold cuts, ham, turkey ham, hot dogs, sausages, sardines, anchovies, pickled herring, or pickled meats; pickled eggs.

Breads & Grains (6 or more servings/day)
- **Allowed:** Enriched white, wheat, rye, and pumpernickel bread; hard rolls, bagels, English muffins, cooked cereal without salt; dry low-sodium cereals; unsalted crackers and breadsticks; corn or flour tortillas; biscuits, muffins, cornbread, pancakes, and waffles all made with low-sodium baking powder; low-sodium or homemade bread crumbs; rice, noodles, barley, spaghetti, macaroni and other pastas; homemade bread stuffing.
- **Avoid:** Breads and rolls with salted tops; quick breads; instant hot cereals; dry cereals with added salt; crackers with salted tops; pancakes, waffles, muffins, biscuits, and cornbread with salt, baking powder, self-rising flour or instant mixes; regular bread crumbs or cracker crumbs; instant rice and pasta mixes; commercial stuffing; commercial casserole mixes.

Vegetables (3 or more servings/day)
- **Allowed:** Fresh, frozen, and low-sodium canned vegetables; regular canned, drained vegetables (limit to ½ cup serving/day); low-sodium vegetable juice; regular vegetable juice (limit ½ cup per day); white or sweet potatoes; salt-free potato chips.
- **Avoid:** Regular canned vegetables (over ½ cup/day); vegetable juices; sauerkraut; pickled vegetables and others prepared in brine; potato casserole mixes; potato chips; frozen vegetables in sauce.

Fruits (3–4 or more servings/day)
- **Allowed:** All fruits and juices.
- **Avoid:** None except salted prunes (saladitos).

Desserts & Sweets
- **Allowed:** Any sweets like sugar, honey, jam, jelly, syrup, marmalade, hard candy; limit regular baked products (e.g., cake, pie, cookies) to 1 serving per day.
- **Avoid:** None.

Beverages
- **Allowed:** Coffee, tea, soft drinks, Postum, alcoholic beverages (if medical approval).
- **Avoid:** Commercially softened water as beverage or in food preparation.

Miscellaneous
- **Allowed:** Limit added salt to ¼ teaspoon per day, may be used in cooking or at the table; limit 3 tsp salted butter or margarine per day; salt-free butter or margarine; vegetable oils, shortening and mayonnaise; salt-free salad dressings; salt substitute with physician's approval; pepper, herbs, and spices; flavorings; vinegar and lemon or lime juice; salt-free seasonings; low-sodium condiments; catsup, chili sauce, mustard, and pickles; fresh-ground horseradish; Tabasco sauce; homemade or salt-free soups; low-sodium baking powder; unsalted snacks: nuts, seeds, pretzels, and popcorn.
- **Avoid:** Added salt in excess of ¼ teaspoon per day; light-salt; garlic salt, celery salt, onion salt, and seasoned salt; sea salt, rock salt, and kosher salt; seasonings containing salt and sodium compounds; monosodium glutamate (MSG, Accent); regular catsup, chili sauce, mustard, pickles, relishes, olives, and horseradish; Kitchen Bouquet; gravy and sauce mixes; barbecue sauce, soy, and teriyaki sauce; Worcestershire and steak sauce; salted snack foods: nuts, seeds, pretzels, and popcorn; commercially prepared convenience foods; regular canned or dried soups.

SAMPLE MENU

Suggested Meal Plan	Suggested Foods and Beverages (may use ¼ teaspoon added salt)
Breakfast Fruit Juice Cereal Meat/Meat Substitute Bread/Margarine Milk Beverage	½ Grapefruit 1 oz. Cornflakes 1 Egg (optional) 2 slices Whole Wheat Toast 1 tsp Margarine* 1 cup 2% Milk* Coffee or Tea
Dinner—Noon or Evening Meal Meat/Meat Substitute Potato/Potato Substitute Vegetable, Salad or Soup Bread/Margarine Dessert Beverage	3 oz Salt-Free Hamburger Patty Salt-Free Oven Fries Tomato Slices & ¼ cup Lettuce 1 cup Salt-Free Vegetable Beef Soup Hamburger Bun 2 Oatmeal Raisin Cookies, ½ cup Fresh Fruit Coffee or Tea
Supper—Evening or Noon Meal Soup or Juice Meat/Meat Substitute Potato/Potato Substitute Vegetable and/or Salad Bread/Margarine Dessert Milk/Beverage	½ cup Salt-Free Tomato Juice 3 oz. Salt-Free Herbed Baked Chicken ½ cup Salt-Free Brown Rice ½ cup Carrot-Raisin Salad/1 tsp dressing 1 slice Whole Wheat Bread/1 tsp Margarine* 4 oz. Strawberry Frozen Yogurt 1 cup 2% Milk*/Coffee or Tea
Snack	½ cup Apple Juice 2 Graham Cracker Squares ½ cup 2% Milk

*To reduce fat in your diet, omit margarine and use 1% or skim milk.

Nutrient Analysis

Calories	2344 Kcal	Riboflavin	2.6 mg
Protein	108 gm	Thiamin	1.7 mg
Carbohydrate	330 gm	Folate	239 mcg
Fat	70 gm	Calcium	1257 mg
Cholesterol	201 mg	Phosphorus	1702 mg
Dietary Fiber	29 gm	Zinc	14 mg
Vitamin A	1812 RE	Iron	15 mg
Vitamin C	248 mg	Sodium	2383 mg
Niacin	32 mg	Potassium	3675 mg

From Griffith HW. Instructions for Patients, 5th ed. Philadelphia, WB Saunders, 1994, pp 539–541. Adapted from Arizona Diet Manual (revised 1992).

PURPOSE

This diet is designed to provide foods containing indigestible fiber as a part of preventive and/or therapeutic nutrition.

DESCRIPTION

The high-fiber diet is based on the basic food groups with a greater emphasis on fiber-rich foods, such as fruits, legumes, vegetables, whole-grain breads, and high-fiber cereals. The Daily Reference Value for fiber is 25 grams (based on 2000 calorie per day diet). The American Diabetes Association has reported that up to 40 gm fiber daily or 25 gm per 1000 Kcal may be beneficial (National Cancer Institute recommends 25–30 gm).

BASIC INFORMATION

Dietary fiber is the component found in many foods that cannot be digested by the intestinal tract. Adequate fluid intake is important when following a high-fiber diet due to the water-binding capacity of fiber. Fiber should be increased in the diet slowly to avoid unpleasant side effects (gas, abdominal bloating/cramps). Dietary fiber can be divided into two separate categories: water-insoluble fiber and water-soluble fiber.

Water Insoluble Fiber

Water insoluble components, such as cellulose, hemicellulose and lignin, remain essentially unchanged during digestion. Foods containing water insoluble fiber include: fruits, vegetables, cereals, and whole grain products. Research suggests that insoluble fiber may be beneficial in the prevention and/or treatment of constipation and diverticular disease and may decrease the risk of colon cancer.

Water-Soluble Fiber

Water-soluble fiber, such as gum, pectin, and mucilages, does dissolve in water and is found in oats, beans, barley, and some fruits and vegetables. Some studies showed that this type of fiber may improve blood glucose and cholesterol levels.

NUTRITIONAL ADEQUACY

The high-fiber diet is adequate in all nutrients. Some studies indicate that excessive consumption of some high-fiber foods may bind and decrease the absorption of the following minerals: calcium, copper, iron, magnesium, selenium, and zinc. However, it is theorized that with a varied, well-balanced diet, mineral or nutrient imbalances are unlikely to happen in those consuming a high-fiber diet.

DIETARY FIBER CONTENT OF FOODS IN COMMONLY SERVED PORTIONS

Food Group	Less 1 gm	1–1.9 gm	2–2.9 gm	3–3.9 gm	4–4.9 gm	5–5.9 gm	6 or more gm
Breads 1 slice	Bagel, white, French	Whole-wheat	bran muffin	None	None	None	None
Cereals 1 oz.	Rice Krispies, Special K, Cornflakes	Oatmeal, Nutri-Grain, Cheerios	Wheaties, Shredded Wheat	Most, Honey Bran	Bran Chex, 40% Bran Flakes, Raisin Bran	Corn Bran	All-Bran, Bran Buds, 100% Bran-Fiber
Pasta 1 cup	None	Macaroni, spaghetti	None	whole-wheat spaghetti	None	None	None
Rice ½ cup	White	Brown	None	None	None	None	None
Legumes ½ cup cooked	None	None	None	Lentils	Lima beans, dried peas	None	Kidney beans, baked beans, navy beans
Vegetables ½ cup	Cucumber, lettuce (1 cup), green pepper	Asparagus, green beans, cabbage, cauliflower, potato (no skin), celery	Broccoli, Brussels sprouts, carrots, corn, potato (with skin), spinach	Peas	None	None	None
Fruits 1 medium	Grapes (20), watermelon (1 cup)	Apricots 3, grapefruit ½, peach with skin, pineapple ½ cup	Apple without skin, banana, orange	Apple with skin, pear with skin, raspberries ½ cup	None	None	None

SAMPLE MENU

Suggested Meal Plan	Suggested Foods and Beverages
Breakfast Fruit Juice Cereal Meat/Meat Substitute Bread/Margarine Milk/Beverage	Prune Juice All Bran Egg Whole Grain Toast & Margarine[*] 1% Milk[*] & Coffee or Tea
Dinner—Noon or Evening Meal Meat/Meat Substitute Potato/Potato Substitute Vegetable and/or Salad Bread/Margarine Dessert Beverage	Meat Loaf Baked Potato Lima Beans, Tossed Salad with Dressing Rye Bread & Margarine[*] Fig Cookie Coffee or Tea
Supper—Evening or Noon Meal Soup or Juice Meat/Meat Substitute Vegetable and/or Salad Bread/Margarine Dessert Milk/Beverage	Lentil Soup Baked Chicken Banana Squash, Tossed Salad & Dressing Rye Bread/Margarine[*] Baked Apple/Cinnamon 1% Milk[*] & Coffee or Tea

[*]To reduce amount of fat in your diet, omit margarine and use skim milk.

Nutrient Analysis

Calories	1930 Kcal	Riboflavin	2.5 mg
Protein	95 gm	Thiamin	1.7 mg
Carbohydrate	239 gm	Folate	527 mcg
Fat	74 gm	Calcium	992 mg
Cholesterol	474 mg	Phosphorus	1789 mg
Dietary Fiber	32 gm	Zinc	15 mg
Vitamin A	2822 RE	Iron	22 mg
Vitamin C	106 mg	Sodium	3180 mg
Niacin	31 mg	Potassium	4158 mg

From Griffith HW. Instructions for Patients, 5th ed. Philadelphia, WB Saunders, 1994, pp 522–523. Adapted from Arizona Diet Manual (revised 1992).

PURPOSE

This diet is designed to eliminate the protein gluten found in wheat, rye, oats, barley, buckwheat, bulgur, or their derivatives for those individuals with gluten-sensitive enteropathy or celiac sprue and dermatitis herpetiformis.

DESCRIPTION

The basic food groups are used as the guide in meal planning. All protein sources are acceptable, except those containing gluten. Products made from the flours or starches of arrowroot, corn, potato, rice, and soybean replace products made from wheat, rye, oats, and barley.

TIPS ON READING LABELS

The following ingredients are frequently listed on product labels. Those from wheat, rye, oat, or barley sources must be excluded from the diet.

Ingredient	Sources Permitted
Hydrolyzed vegetable protein (HVP) or texturized or vegetable protein (TVP)	Soy or corn
Flour or cereal products	Rice, corn, potato, or soy
Vegetable protein	Soy or corn
Malt or malt flavoring	Corn only
Starch	Cornstarch only
Modified starch or modified food starch	Arrowroot, corn, potato, tapioca, maize
Vegetable gum	Carob or locust bean: cellulose or sugar gum; gum acacia, arabic tragacanth or xanthin
Soy sauce, soy sauce solids	Without wheat

NUTRITIONAL ADEQUACY

This diet should be adequate in all nutrients. An added effort will need to be made to ensure adequate fiber.

FOOD LISTS

Food Groups	Foods Allowed	Foods to Avoid
Breads/Grains	Corn flakes, cornmeal, hominy, rice, puffed rice, Cream of Rice, Rice Krispies. Made from rice, corn, soybean flour or gluten free wheat starch, arrowroot, tapioca, gluten free wheat starch. Homemade broth, vegetable, or cream soups made w/ allowed ingredients.	Wheat, rye, oatmeal, barley, wheat germ, kasha, macaroni, noodles, spaghetti, crackers, chips, cereals containing malt flavorings, buckwheat, bran, or bulgur. Prepared cake, bread, pancake, or waffle mixes. Any made with wheat, rye, barley, or oats. Commercially prepared soups made with wheat, rye, oats, or barley products; broth, bouillon, and soup mixes.
Fruits/Vegetables	All except items listed to avoid.	Any thickened or prepared (i.e., some pie fillings). Any creamed or breaded vegetables.
Milk/Dairy	All except items listed to avoid.	Commercial chocolate milk w/cereal addition. Malted milk. Instant milk drinks. Hot cocoa mixes. Nondairy cream substitutes. Processed cheese, cheese foods, and spreads containing a gluten source. Cheese containing oat gum.
Meat/Meat Substitutes	Any plain products, including eggs.	Any prepared with stabilizers or fillers, such as frankfurters, luncheon meats, sandwich spreads, sausages, and canned meats; breaded fish or meats. Poultry prepared with hydrolyzed or texturized vegetable protein (HVP, TVP). Read labels.
Desserts/Sweets	Gelatin desserts, ices, homemade ice cream, custard, junket, rice pudding. Cakes, cookies, and pastries prepared with gluten-free wheat starch. Syrup, jelly, jam, hard candies, molasses, and marshmallows.	All others unless labeled gluten-free. Read labels.
Beverages	Carbonated beverages, fruit juices, tea, coffee, decaffeinated coffee to which no wheat flour has been added.	Postum, Ovaltine, ale, beer, root beer.
Miscellaneous	Herbs, spices, pickles, vinegar, syrups, sugar, popcorn, molasses, potato chips, jelly, jam, honey, corn syrup. Butter or fortified margarine.	Commercial salad dressings, except pure mayonnaise (read labels). Any foods prepared w/wheat, rye, oats, barley, and buckwheat, some catsup, chili sauce, soy sauce, mustard, horseradish, some dry seasoning mixes, pickles, distilled white vinegar, steak sauce, stabilizers, sauces and gravies w/gluten sources, some chewing gum, chip dips, malt or malt flavoring, unless derived from corn, baking powder.

SAMPLE MENU

Suggested Meal Plan	Suggested Foods and Beverages
Breakfast Fruit Juice Cereal Meat/Meat Substitute Bread/Margarine Milk Beverage	Apricot Nectar Cream of Rice Poached Egg Rice Cake 2% Milk[*] Coffee
Dinner—Noon or Evening Meal Meat/Meat Substitute Potato/Potato Substitute Vegetable and/or Salad Bread/Margarine Dessert Beverage	3 oz. Beef Patty (no fillers) Mashed Potato Frozen Peas, Sliced Tomato Salad 2 slices Gluten-Free Bread Fresh Apple Coffee
Supper—Evening or Noon Meal Soup or Juice Meat/Meat Substitute Potato/Potato Substitute Vegetable and/or Salad Bread/Margarine Dessert Milk/Beverage	Tomato Juice Baked Chicken Rice, Spinach, Fruited Gelatin Salad Corn Tortilla Rice Pudding 2% Milk,[*] Coffee

[*]To reduce amount of fat in your diet, use 1% or skim milk.

Nutrient Analysis

Calories	1939 Kcal	Riboflavin	12.0 mg
Protein	96 gm	Thiamin	1.3 mg
Carbohydrate	257 gm	Folate	315 mcg
Fat	62 gm	Calcium	1073 mg
Cholesterol	457 mg	Phosphorus	1374 mg
Dietary Fiber	17 gm	Zinc	11 mg
Vitamin A	2619 RE	Iron	14 mg
Vitamin C	158 mg	Sodium	1877 mg
Niacin	24.5 mg	Potassium	3384 mg

From Griffith HW. Instructions for Patients, 5th ed. Philadelphia, WB Saunders, 1994, pp 524–525. Adapted from Arizona Diet Manual (revised 1992).

PURPOSE

This diet is designed to minimize gastrointestinal (GI) disturbances associated with ingestion of the carbohydrate lactose, such as abdominal cramps, bloating, flatulence, increased GI motility, and diarrhea.

DESCRIPTION

This diet is individualized to provide the appropriate amount of lactose that a lactose-intolerant individual may tolerate. Milk and milk products are limited.

BASIC INFORMATION

Current research indicates that most lactose-intolerant individuals can consume 15 to 30 grams of lactose without experiencing severe symptoms. Tolerance level is highly individualized.

NUTRITIONAL ADEQUACY

This diet may provide adequate amounts of essential nutrients based on the use of lactose-reduced food choices. If lactose-reduced foods are not included, the diet may be deficient in calcium, vitamin D, or riboflavin.

FOOD LISTS

Food Groups	Foods Allowed	Foods to Avoid
Milk/Dairy	Milk substitutes and nondairy products. Milk treated with lactose reducing enzymes.	Milk or milk products in excess of allowed amounts. Avoid or decrease intake with development of intolerance.
Meats/Meat Substitutes	Any meat, fish, and poultry, except those listed to avoid, peanut butter. The following cheeses contain no detectable lactose and may be used if tolerated—brick, Swiss, Camembert, cheddar, Colby, mozzarella, muenster, provolone. Eggs without milk.	All other cheeses and cheese products. Creamed meats. Casseroles made with foods to avoid. Breaded meats, fish, or poultry. Eggs made with milk, souffles, quiche with milk or cream.
Breads/Grains	Breads, cereals, crackers. Quick breads (muffins, biscuits, etc.) in moderation, if made with milk. Broth-type soups.	Excessive use of commercial products with added milk or lactose. Milk- or cream-based soups.
Fruits/ Vegetables	Any fresh, canned, or frozen.	Artificial fruit juice containing lactose and dietetic fruits with added lactose. Creamed vegetables or vegetables in cheese sauce.
Desserts/ Sweets	Sugar, honey, jelly, jams. Plain sugar candies, such as gumdrops, jelly beans, marshmallows. Angel food cake, fruit ices, gelatin. Commercial mixes or baked products containing milk in moderation. Nondairy frozen desserts.	Cream candies, tablet candies containing lactose. Cream pies. Products with cream fillings, cream cheese, or sour cream. Commercial puddings.
Beverages	Coffee, tea, carbonated beverages, cereal beverages, alcoholic beverages, if allowed by physician. Isomil, Pregestimil, ProSobee.	Cocoa, Ovaltine, cocoa malt, cocoa mixes, beverages containing cream.
Miscellaneous	Condiments, pure flavorings, popcorn, nuts, salt, vinegar, spices, lactate, lactic acid, lactalbumin, citric acid, MSG, margarine, butter, bacon, lard, mayonnaise, vegetable oils, vegetable shortenings. Most oil-based commercial salad dressing. Nondairy whipped cream.	Cream sauces, milk gravies, gum ascorbic acid tablets, spice blends with lactose added, peppermints, whey. Salad dressing with added milk or cheese. Sour cream, alone, or in spreads and dips, cream cheese, whipped cream, milk gravies.

SAMPLE MENU

Suggested Meal Plan	Suggested Foods and Beverages
Breakfast Fruit Juice Cereal Meat/Meat Substitute Bread/Margarine Milk Beverage	Orange Juice w/Calcium Shredded Wheat Soft Cooked Egg Wheat Toast/Margarine Lactose-Free Milk Coffee
Dinner—Noon or Evening Meal Meat/Meat Substitute Potato/Potato Substitute Vegetable and/or Salad Bread/Margarine Dessert Beverage	Baked Chicken Brown Rice Spinach, Sliced Tomato Salad Wheat Bread/Margarine Angel Food Cake, Strawberries Coffee
Supper—Evening or Noon Meal Soup or Juice Meat/Meat Substitute Vegetable and/or Salad Bread/Margarine Dessert Beverage	Apple Juice Lean Roast Beef Cooked Carrots, Three Bean Salad Rye Bread Fruit Sorbet Coffee or Tea

Nutrient Analysis

Calories	1843 Kcal	Riboflavin	1.5 mg
Protein	90 gm	Thiamin	1.4 mg
Carbohydrate	250 gm	Folate	325 mcg
Fat	59 gm	Calcium	(varies) mg
Cholesterol	373 mg	Phosphorus	1112 mg
Dietary Fiber	7 gm	Zinc	11 mg
Vitamin A	2941 RE	Iron	22 mg
Vitamin C	152 mg	Sodium	1637 mg
Niacin	24 mg	Potassium	2763 mg

From Griffith HW. Instructions for Patients, 5th ed. Philadelphia, WB Saunders, 1994, pp 527–528. Adapted from Arizona Diet Manual (revised 1992).

Weight-Reduction Diet 800 Calories (approximately)	Carbohydrate: 75 g Protein: 55 g Fat: 30 g

Breakfast

1 fruit exchange (List 3)	Orange juice. . . . . ½ cup
1 bread exchange (List 4)	Toast . . . . 1 slice
1 meat exchange (List 5)	Egg 1
1 fat exchange (List 6)	Margarine . . . . 1 tsp
½ cup skim milk (List 1)	Skim milk . . . . ½ cup

Lunch

2 meat exchanges (List 5)	Cheese . . . . 2 1-oz. slices
1 vegetable exchange (List 2)	Tomatoes . . . . ½ cup
Vegetable(s) as desired (List 2*)	Lettuce, etc . . . . as desired
1 fruit exchange (List 3)	Apple . . . . 1 small
½ cup skim milk (List 1)	Skim milk . . . . ½ cup
	Low-calorie dressing . . . . 1 Tbsp

Dinner

2 meat exchanges (List 5)	Chicken, baked . . . . 2 oz
1 vegetable exchange (List 2)	Broccoli . . . . ½ cup
Vegetable(s) as desired (List 2*)	Lettuce, etc. . . . . as desired
1 fruit exchange (List 3)	Orange . . . . 1 small
½ cup skim milk (List 1)	Skim milk . . . . ½ cup

Instructions for Daily Menu Guide

The foods allowed in your diet should be selected from the exchange lists. Menus should be planned on the basis of the daily menu guide. Foods in the same list are interchangeable, because, in the quantities specified, they provide approximately the same amounts of carbohydrate, protein, and fat. For example, when your menu calls for one bread exchange, any item in List 4 may be used in the amount stated. If two bread exchanges are allowed, double the specified amount or use a single exchange of *two* foods in List 4. A day's sample menus are given to illustrate correct use of the exchange lists.

The most success will be achieved if all of the foods allotted in this plan are eaten. For best results, do not skip any meals, and do not save any uneaten portions for the next day. Remember that ideal body weight is achieved when energy taken in is equal to energy output.

Foods Allowed in Reasonable Amounts

Seasonings: Celery salt, cinnamon, garlic, garlic or onion salt, horseradish, lemon, mint, mustard, nutmeg, parsley, pepper, noncaloric sweeteners, spices, vanilla, and vinegar.

Other Foods: Coffee or tea (no sugar or cream), diet beverage without sugar, fat-free broth, bouillon, unflavored gelatin, artificially sweetened fruit-flavored gelatin, sour or dill pickles, and cranberries or rhubarb (without sugar).

List 1 Milk Values

Each portion supplies approximately 12 gm of carbohydrate and 8 gm of protein; the fat content and total calories vary with the type of milk. (One fat exchange equals 5 gm of fat.)

	measurement	fat exchanges	calories
Milk			
Buttermilk	1 cup	—	80
Evaporated, undiluted			
Skim	½ cup	½	80
Whole	½ cup	2	170
Nonfat dry milk mixed according to directions on box	1 cup	—	80
Nonfat dry milk powder	1 cup	—	80
Skim	1 cup	—	80
1% butterfat	1 cup	½	107
2% butterfat	1 cup	1	125
Whole	1 cup	2	170
Yogurt, plain made with skim milk	1 cup	—	80

If substitution for the milk indicated in the diet plan is desired, choose either a milk product that contains the same number of fat exchanges or allow for the difference in the meal plan. For example, if the diet plan calls for 1 cup of skim milk (no fat exchange), substitute 1 cup of 2% milk by omitting one fat exchange.

List 2 Vegetable Exchanges

Each portion (except for vegetables marked with an *) supplies approximately 5 gm of carbohydrate and 2 gm of protein, or 25 calories. One serving equals ½ cup.

Asparagus	*Lettuce
Beans, green or yellow	Mushrooms
Bean sprouts	Okra
Beets	Onions
Broccoli	*Parsley
Brussels sprouts	Peppers, green or red
Cabbage	*Radishes
Carrots	Rutabagas
Cauliflower	Sauerkraut
Celery	Squash, summer
*Chicory	Tomatoes
*Chinese cabbage	Tomato juice
Cucumbers	Turnips
Eggplant	Vegetable juice cocktail
*Endive	*Watercress
*Endive	Zucchini
*Escarole	
Greens: beet, chard, collard, dandelion, kale, mustard, spinach, turnip	

*May be used as desired.

List 3 Fruit Exchanges

(fresh, dried, frozen, or canned without sugar or syrup)
Each portion supplies approximately 10 gm of carbohydrate, or 40 calories.

	measurement
Apple	1 small (2-in. diam.)
Apple juice or cider	1 cup
Applesauce	½ cup
Apricots, fresh	2 med.
Apricots, dried	4 halves
Banana	½ small
Berries (boysenberries, blackberries, blueberries, raspberries)	½ cup
Cantaloupe	¼ (6-in. diam.)
Cherries	10 large
Dates	2
Figs, fresh	1 large
Figs, dried	1 small
Fruit cocktail	½ cup
Grapefruit	½ small
Grapefruit juice	½ cup
Grapes	12
Grape juice	¼ cup
Honeydew melon	⅛ (7-in. diam.)
Mandarin oranges	¾ cup
Mango	½ small
Nectarine	1 small
Orange	1 small
Orange juice	½ cup
Papaya	¾ cup
Peach	1 med.
Pear	1 small
Persimmon, native	1 med.
Pineapple	½ cup
Pineapple juice	1 cup
Plums	2 med.
Prunes	2 med.
Prune juice	¼ cup
Raisins	2 Tbsp
Strawberries	¾ cup
Tangerine	1 large
Watermelon	1 cup

List 4 Bread Exchanges

Each portion supplies approximately 15 gm of carbohydrate and 2 gm of protein, or 79 calories.

	measurement
Bread, French, raisin (without icing) rye, white, whole-wheat	1 slice
Bagel	½
Biscuit, roll	1 (2-in. diam.)
Bun (for hamburger or wiener)	½
Cornbread	1 in. × 2 in. × 2 in.
English muffin	½
Muffin	1 (2-in. diam.)
¹⁄₂₀ Cake, angel or sponge, without icing	1 ½-in. cube (of 10-in.–diam. cake)
Cereal, cooked	½ cup
Dry (flaked or puffed)	¾ cup

Cornstarch ....2 Tbsp

Crackers, graham ....2 (2 ½-in. sq)

    Oyster ....20 (½ cup)

    Round 6

    Rye wafer...3 (2 in. × 3½ in.)

    Saltine 6

    Variety ....5 small

Flour ....2 ½ Tbsp

Matzo ....1 (6-in. diam.)

Popcorn, popped, unbuttered,

    small-kernel ....1 ½ cups

Pretzels (3-ring) 6

Rice or grits, cooked..½ cup

Spaghetti, macaroni, noodles, cooked ....½ cup

Tortilla ....1 (6-in. diam.)

Vegetables

Beans, baked, without pork ....¼ cup

    Lima, navy, etc., dry, cooked ....½ cup

Corn...⅓ cup

    Corn on the cob...................................½ med. Ear

Parsnips ....⅔ cup

Peas, dried (split peas, etc.) or

    green, cooked ....½ cup

Potatoes, sweet, or yams, fresh..........................¼ cup

    White, baked or boiled.........................1 (2-in. diam.)

    White, mashed...½ cup

Pumpkin ....¾ cup

Squash, winter (acorn or butternut) ....½ cup

Wheat germ ....¼ cup

List **5** Meat Exchanges

Each portion supplies approximately 7 gm of protein and
5 gm of fat, or 73 calories.

                                     measurement

Cheese, cheddar,

    American, Swiss...1-oz. slice

                (3½-in. sq, ⅛-in. thick)

    Cottage ....¼ cup

Egg 1

Fish and seafood

    Halibut, perch, sole, etc. ....1-oz. slice

                   (4 in. × 2 in. × ¼ in.)

    Oysters, clams, shrimp, scallops ....5 small

    Salmon, tuna, crab..¼ cup

    Sardines ....3 med.

Meat and poultry

    Beef, lamb, pork, veal, ham,

        liver, chicken, etc. (med. Fat) ....1-oz. slice

                   (4 in. × 2 in. × ¼ in.)

    Cold cuts ....1 ½-oz. slice

              (4½ in. sq. ⅛-in. thick)

    Vienna sausages..2

    † Wiener ....1 (10 per lb.)

Peanut butter (omit two

    additional fat exchanges) ....2 Tbsp

_____

† Limit wieners to one exchange per day.

List **6** Fat Exchanges

Each portion supplies approximately 5 gm of fat, or 45
calories.

                                     measurement

Avocado ....¼ (4-in. diam.)

Bacon, crisp..1 slice

Butter or margarine ....1 tsp

Cream, half-and-half..3 Tbsp

    Heavy, 40%..1 Tbsp

    Light, 20%..2 Tbsp

    Sour ....2 Tbsp

Cream cheese...1 Tbsp

Dressing, French...1 Tbsp

    Italian..1 Tbsp

    Mayonnaise...1 tsp

    Mayonnaise-type...2 tsp

    Roquefort ....2 tsp

Nuts...6 small

Oil or cooking fat ....1 tsp

Olives ....5 small

Adapted from Eli Lilly and Company, Indianapolis, Indiana 46286.

Daily Menu Guide/1000 Calories (approximately)

Carbohydrate: 125 gm
Protein: 50 gm
Fat: 35 gm

Breakfast

1 fruit exchange (List 3)
1 ½ bread exchanges (List 4)
1 meat exchange (List 5)
1 fat exchange (List 6)
½ cup skim milk (List 1)

Breakfast

Orange juice.................................. ½ cup
Cereal, cooked......................*EXAMPLE*................. ¾ cup
Egg.. 1
Margarine .... 1 tsp
Skim milk...................................... ½ cup

Lunch

1 meat exchange (List 5)
1 ½ bread exchanges (List 4)
Vegetable(s) as desired (List 2*)
1 fruit exchange List 3)
1 fat exchange (List 6)
½ cup skim milk (List 1)

Lunch

Cheese .... 1-oz. slice
Rye wafers 5
Lettuce, etc. ....*EXAMPLE*........ as desired
Apple..................*EXAMPLE*.............. 1 small
French dressing............................. 1 Tbsp
Skim milk..................................... ½ cup

Dinner

2 meat exchanges (List 5)
1 bread exchange (List 4)
1 vegetable exchange (List 2)
Vegetable(s), as desired (List 2*)
1 fruit exchange (List 3)
1 fat exchange (List 6)
½ cup skim milk (List 1)

Dinner

Chicken, baked............................. 2 oz.
Peas... ½ cup
Tomatoes .... ½ cup
Lettuce, etc. ....*EXAMPLE*........ as desired
Fruit cocktail ....*EXAMPLE*............ ½ cup
Margarine ....1 tsp
Skim milk...................................... ½ cup

Bedtime Snack

½ bread exchange (List 4)
½ cup skim milk (List 1)

Bedtime Snack

Graham cracker ....*EXAMPLE*............ 1 square
Skim milk.........*EXAMPLE*................. ½ cup

Foods Allowed in Reasonable Amounts

Seasonings: Celery salt, cinnamon, garlic, garlic or onion salt, horseradish, lemon, mint, mustard, nutmeg, parsley, pepper, noncaloric sweeteners, spices, vanilla, and vinegar.

Other Foods: Coffee or tea (no sugar or cream), diet beverage without sugar, fat-free broth, bouillon, unflavored gelatin, artificially sweetened fruit-flavored gelatin, sour or dill pickles, and cranberries or rhubarb (without sugar).

List 1 Milk Values

Each portion supplies approximately 12 gm of carbohydrate and 8 gm of protein; the fat content and total calories vary with the type of milk. (One fat exchange equals 5 gm of fat.)

	measurement	fat exchanges	calories
Milk			
Buttermilk	1 cup	—	80
Evaporated, undiluted			
Skim	½ cup	—	80
Whole	½ cup	2	170
Nonfat dry milk mixed according to directions on box	1 cup	—	80
Nonfat dry milk powder	a cup	—	80
Skim	1 cup	—	80
1% butterfat	1 cup	½	107
2% butterfat	1 cup	1	125
Whole	1 cup	2	170
Yogurt, plain, made with skim milk	1 cup	—	80

If substitution for the milk indicated in the diet plan is desired, choose either a milk product that contains the same number of fat exchanges or allow for the difference in the meal plan. For example, if the diet plan calls for 1 cup of skim milk (no fat exchange), substitute 1 cup of 2% milk by omitting one fat exchange.

List 2 Vegetable Exchanges

Each portion (except for vegetables marked with an *) supplies approximately 5 gm of carbohydrate and 2 gm of protein, or 25 calories. One serving equals ½ cup.

Asparagus	*Lettuce
Beans, green or yellow	Mushrooms
Bean sprouts	Okra
Beets	Onions
Broccoli	*Parsley
Brussels sprouts	Peppers, green or red
Cabbage	*Radishes
Carrots	Rutabagas
Cauliflower	Sauerkraut
Celery	Squash, summer
*Chicory	Tomatoes
*Chinese cabbage	Tomato juice

Cucumbers
Eggplant
*Endive
*Escarole
Greens: beet, chard, collard,
    dandelion, kale, mustard,
    spinach, turnip

Turnips
Vegetable juice cocktail
*Watercress
Zucchini

---

*May be used as desired.

List 3 Fruit Exchanges

(fresh, dried, or frozen or canned without sugar or syrup)
Each portion supplies approximately 10 gm of carbohydrates, or 40 calories.

	measurement
Apple	1 small (2-in. diam.)
Apple juice or cider	1 cup
Applesauce	½ cup
Apricots, fresh	2 med.
Apricots, dried	4 halves
Banana	½ small
Berries (boysenberries, blackberries, blueberries, raspberries)	½ cup
Cantaloupe	¼ (6-in. diam.)
Cherries	10 large
Dates	2
Figs, fresh	1 large
Figs, dried	1 small
Fruit cocktail	½ cup
Grapefruit	½ small
Grapefruit juice	½ cup
Grapes	12
Grape juice	¼ cup
Honeydew melon	⅛ (7-in. diam.)
Mandarin oranges	¾ cup
Mango	½ small
Nectarine	1 small
Orange	1 small
Orange juice	½ cup
Papaya	¾ cup
Peach	1 med.
Pear	1 small
Persimmon, native	1 med.
Pineapple	½ cup
Pineapple juice	⅓ cup
Plums	2 med.
Prunes	2 med.
Prune juice	¼ cup
Raisins	2 Tbsp
Strawberries	¾ cup
Tangerine	1 large
Watermelon	1 cup

List 4 Bread Exchanges

Each portion supplies approximately 15 gm of
carbohydrate and 2 gm of protein, or 70 calories.

	measurement
Bread, French, raisin (without icing), rye, white, whole-wheat	1 slice
Bagel	½
Biscuit, roll	1 (2-in. diam.)
Bread crumbs, dried	3 Tbsp
Bun (for hamburger or wiener)	½
Cornbread	1 in. × 2 in. × 2 in.
English muffin	½
Muffin	1 (2-in. diam.)
⅟20 Cake, angel or sponge, without icing	1 ½-in. cube (of 10-in.–diam. cake)
Cereal, cooked	½ cup
Dry (flaked or puffed)	¾ cup
Cornstarch	2 Tbsp
Crackers, graham	2 (2½-in. sq)
Oyster	20 (½ cup)
Round	6
Rye wafer	3 (2 in. × 3½ in.)
Saltine	6
Variety	5 small
Flour	2 ½ Tbsp
Matzo	1 (6-in. diam.)
Popcorn, popped, unbuttered, small-kernel	1½ cups
Pretzels (3-ring)	6
Rice or grits, cooked	½ cup
Spaghetti, macaroni, noodles, cooked	½ cup
Tortilla	1 (6-in. diam.)
Vegetables	
Beans, baked, without pork	¼ cup
Lima, navy, etc., dry, cooked	½ cup
Corn	⅓ cup
Corn on the cob	½ med. ear
Parsnips	⅔ cup
Peas, dried (split peas, etc.) or green, cooked	½ cup
Potatoes, sweet, or Yams, fresh	¼ cup
White, baked or boiled	1 (2-in. diam.)
White, mashed	½ cup
Pumpkin	¾ cup
Squash, winter (acorn or butternut)	½ cup
Wheat germ	¼ cup

List 5 Meat Exchanges

Each portion supplies approximately 7 gm of protein and
5 gm of fat, or 73 calories.

	measurement
Cheese, cheddar, American, Swiss	1-oz slice (3½-in. sq, ⅛-in. thick)
Cottage	¼ cup

Daily Menu Guide/1000 Calories (approximately)

Egg 1

Fish and seafood

   Halibut, perch,

      sole, etc. . . . . 1-oz slice (4 in. × 2 in. × ¼ in.)

   Oysters, clams, shrimp,

      scallops. . . . . 5 small

   Salmon, tuna, crab. . . . . ¼ cup

   Sardines . . . . 3 med.

Meat and poultry

   Beef, lamb, pork, veal, ham,

     liver, chicken, etc.

     (med. fat) . . . . 1-oz slice (4 in. × 2 in. × ¼ in.)

   Cold cuts. . . . . 1½-oz slice (4½-in. sq, ⅛-in. thick)

   Vienna sausages. 2

   †Wiener . . . . 1 (10 per lb)

Peanut butter (omit two additional

   fat exchanges) . . . . 2 Tbsp

---

†Limit wieners to one exchange per day.

List 6 Fat Exchanges

Each portion supplies approximately 5 gm of fat, or 45 calories.

	measurement
Avocado	⅛ (4-in. diam.)
Bacon, crisp	1 slice
Butter or margarine	1 tsp
Cream, half-and-half.	3 Tbsp
Heavy, 40%	1 Tbsp
Light, 20%	2 Tbsp
Sour.	2 Tbsp

Cream cheese.	1 Tbsp
Dressing, French	1 Tbsp
Italian	1 Tbsp
Mayonnaise	1 tsp
Mayonnaise-type.	2 tsp
Roquefort	2 tsp
Nuts.	6 small
Oil or cooking fat.	1 tsp
Olives	5 small

Miscellaneous Foods

The following foods may be used, if you wish, but they must be figured into the daily diet plan, with the food exchanges allowed as indicated.

	measurement	exchange
Fish sticks, frozen	3 sticks	1 bread, 2 meat
Fruit-flavored gelatin	¼ cup	1 bread
Ginger ale	7 oz	1 bread
Ice cream, vanilla, chocolate, strawberry	½ cup	1 bread, 2 fat
Low-calorie dressing, French or Italian	1 Tbsp	— ‡
Potato or corn chips	10 larger or 15 small	1 bread, 2 fat
Sherbet	½ cup	2 bread
Vanilla wafers	6	1 bread
Waffle, frozen	1 (5½ in.)	1 bread, 1 fat

---

‡The fat and calorie contents do not have to be counted if the amount is limited to 1 tablespoonful.

Adapted from Eli Lilly and Company, Indianapolis, Indiana 46286.

Carbohydrate: 164 gm
Protein: 54 gm
Fat: 37 gm

Daily Menu Guide/1200 Calories

Breakfast
1 Fruit (List 4)	½ cup orange juice
2 Starch/bread (List 1)	2 slices whole wheat toast
1 Fat (List 6)	1 tsp margarine
1 Milk (List 5)	1 cup 1% milk
*Free foods (List 7)	Coffee or tea

Lunch
1 Meat (List 2)	¼ cup tuna
1 Starch/bread (List 1)	1 slice rye bread
1 Fruit (List 4)	½ banana
1 Fat (List 6)	2 tsp salad dressing, mayonnaise-type
*Free foods (List 7)	¼ cup chopped celery

Afternoon Snack
1 Fruit (List 4)	1 small apple

Dinner
2 Meat (List 2)	2 oz. roast beef
1 Starch/bread (List 1)	1 small potato
1 Vegetable (List 3)	½ cup broccoli
1 Fruit (List 4)	1¼ cup strawberries
1 Fat (List 6)	1 tsp margarine
*Free foods (List 7)	salad greens, radishes, 2 Tbsp low-calorie salad dressing

Evening Snack
1 Starch/Bread (List 1)	3 graham crackers
1 Milk (List 5)	1 cup 1% milk

*Choose no more than three portions daily of those items that have a serving size given on the FREE FOOD LISTS

1 Starches and Breads

One portion of each food in this list contains about 15 gm carbohydrate, 3 gm protein, a trace of fat, and 80 calories.

To choose a similar portion of a starch or bread not listed, follow these general rules:

• Cereal, grain, pasta—½ cup
• Bread product—1 oz.

Breads

	Portion
Bagel	½ (1 oz.)
Bun (hamburger, hot dog)	½ (1 oz.)
English muffin	½
Pita (6 in. across)	½
Tortilla, flour or corn (6 in. across)	1
Whole wheat, rye, white, pumpernickel, raisin (no icing)	1 slice (1 oz.)

Cereals/Grains/Pasta

Bran cereal, concentrated, such as Bran Buds, All-Bran	1 cup
Bran cereal, flaked	½ cup
Cooked cereal, grits, bulgur	½ cup
Grape-Nuts	3 Tbsp
Macaroni, noodles, spaghetti (cooked)	½ cup
Puffed cereal	1½ cup
Ready-to-eat cereal, unsweetened	¾ cup
Rice, white or brown	1 cup
Shredded wheat	⅓ cup
Wheat germ	3 Tbsp

Crackers/Snacks

Graham cracker (2½-in. square)	3
Matzo	¾ oz.
Melba toast	5 slices
Oyster crackers	24

Daily Menu Guide/1200 Calories

Popcorn, popped, no fat added	3 cups
Pretzels	¾ oz.
Ry Krisp (2 in. × 3½ in.)	4

Starchy Vegetables

Beans, baked	¼ cup
Corn	½ cup or 6-in. cob
Lentils, beans, or peas (dried), such as kidney, white, split, black-eyed	1 cup
Lima beans	½ cup
Peas, green (canned or frozen)	½ cup
Potato, baked	1 small (3 oz.)
Potato, mashed	⅓ cup
Winter squash (acorn, butternut)	¾ cup
Yam or sweet potato, plain	1 cup

Starch Foods Prepared with Fat

(Count as 1 starch/bread exchange and 1 fat exchange)

Biscuit (2½ in. across)	1
Chow mein noodles	½ cup
Corn bread (2-in. cube)	1 (2 oz.)
Cracker, round butter type	6
French fried potatoes (2–3½ in. long)	10 (1½ oz.)
Muffin (small, plain)	1
Taco shell (6 in. across)	2

 Meats and Meat Substitutes

One portion of each food in this list contains about 7 gm protein. Lean meats and meat substitutes have about 55 calories per serving; other meat items have 78 to 100 calories per serving. To follow a diet low in cholesterol and saturated fat, choose the lean meats, fish, and other items that appear in bold type. Portions are weighed after cooking and with skin, bones, and fat removed.

	Portion

Beef

Lean cuts, such as USDA Good/ Choice round, sirloin, or flank steak, tenderloin, chipped beef	1 oz.
All other cuts	1 oz.

Cheese

Cottage or ricotta	¼ cup
Diet (less than 55 calories per oz.)	1 oz.
Parmesan, grated	2 Tbsp
Other cheese (except cream cheese)	1 oz.

Eggs

Egg substitute (less than 55 calories per ¼ cup)	¼ cup
Egg white*	3
Egg, whole*	1

Fish and Seafood

All fresh or frozen fish	1 oz.
Clams, crab, lobster, shrimp, scallops	2 oz.
Herring, smoked	1 oz.
Oysters	6 medium
Sardines (canned)	2 medium
Tuna (water-packed)	¼ cup
Salmon (canned)	¼ cup

Miscellaneous

Hot dog† (10 per lb)	1
Lamb (all cuts)	1 oz.
Liver,* heart,* kidney,* sweet breads*	1 oz.
Luncheon meats—**95% fat free;** all others	1 oz.
Peanut butter	1 Tbsp
Sausages, such as Polish, Italian, smoked	1 oz.

Pork

Lean cuts, such as **Canadian bacon; fresh ham; canned, cured, boiled ham; tenderloin**	1 oz.
Other cuts	1 oz.

Poultry

Chicken, turkey, Cornish hen (skin removed)	1 oz.

Veal

Lean chops and roasts	1 oz.
Cutlets	1 oz.

3 Vegetables

One portion of each vegetable in this list contains about 5 gm carbohydrate, 2 gm protein, and 25 calories. If no portion size is listed, the following measurements should be used:

• Cooked vegetables or juice—½ cup
• Raw vegetables—1 cup

Check Free Foods (List 7) and Starches/Breads (List 1) for vegetables not listed here.

Asparagus
Beans (green, wax, Italian)
Bean sprouts
Beets
Broccoli
Brussels sprouts
Cabbage (cooked)
Carrots
Cauliflower
Eggplant
Greens (collard, mustard, etc.)
Mushrooms (cooked)
Okra
Onion
Peapods (snow peas)
Peppers (green)
Sauerkraut
Spinach (cooked)
Summer squash (crookneck)
Tomato (1 large)
Tomato or vegetable juice
Turnip
Water chestnuts
Zucchini (cooked)

4 Fruits

One portion of each fruit here contains about 15 gm carbohydrate and 60 calories. To choose a similar portion of a fruit not listed, follow these general rules:
- Fresh, canned, or frozen fruit, no sugar added—½ cup
- Dried fruit—¼

	Portion
Apple, raw (2 in. across)	1
Applesauce, no sugar added	½ cup
Apricot, raw (medium)	4
Banana (9 in. long)	½
Blackberries or blueberries, raw	¼ cup
Cantaloupe or honeydew melon	1 cup
Cherries, raw (large)	12
Fig, raw (2 in. across)	2
Fruit cocktail, canned	½ cup
Grapefruit (medium)	½
Grapefruit segments	¾ cup
Grapes (small)	15
Kiwi (large)	1
Mandarin orange	¾ cup
Nectarine (2½ in. across)	1
Orange (2½ in. across)	1
Papaya	1 cup
Peach (2¾ in. across)	1 whole or ¾ cup
Pear	½ large or 1 small
Persimmon (native, medium)	2
Pineapple, fresh	¾ cup
Pineapple, canned	1 cup
Plum, raw (2 in. across)	2
Raspberries, raw	1 cup
Strawberries, raw (whole)	1¼ cup
Tangerine (2½ in. across)	2
Watermelon	1¼ cup

Dried Fruits

Apple	4 rings
Apricot	7 halves
Date (medium)	2½
Fig	1½
Prune (medium)	3
Raisins	2 Tbsp

Fruit Juices

Apple juice or cider	½ cup
Cranberry juice cocktail	1 cup
Grape juice	1 cup
Prune juice	1 cup
Other, such as orange, pineapple, etc.	½ cup

5 Milk and Milk Products

One portion of each milk or milk product on this list contains about 12 gm carbohydrate and 8 gm protein. These foods also contain 1 to 8 gm fat and 90 to 150 calories per serving, depending on their butterfat content. Choose foods from the skim and lowfat milk groups as often as possible, because they contain less butterfat than do whole milk products.

Skim and Very Lowfat Milk

Skim, ½%, or 1% milk	1 cup
Buttermilk, lowfat	1 cup
Evaporated skim milk	½ cup
Nonfat dry milk	1 cup
Nonfat yogurt, plain	8 oz.

Lowfat Milk
(Count as 1 milk exchange and 1 fat exchange)

2% milk	1 cup
Lowfat yogurt, plain (with added nonfat milk solids)	8 oz.

Whole Milk
(Count as 1 milk exchange and 2 fat exchanges)

Whole milk	1 cup
Evaporated whole milk	½ cup
Whole yogurt, plain	8 oz.

6 Fats

One portion of each food on this list contains about 5 gm fat and 45 calories. Choose unsaturated fats instead of saturated fats as often as possible.

Unsaturated Fats	Portion
Almonds, dry roasted	6 whole
Avocado (medium)	⅛
Margarine	1 tsp
Margarine, diet	1 Tbsp
Mayonnaise	1 tsp
Oil (corn, cottonseed, olive, peanut, safflower, soybean, sunflower)	1 tsp
Olives	10 small or 5 large
Peanuts	20 small or 10 large
Pecans or walnuts	2 whole
Salad dressing, mayonnaise-type	2 tsp
Salad dressing, other varieties	1 Tbsp
Sunflower seeds	1 Tbsp

Saturated Fats	
Bacon	1 slice
Butter	1 tsp
Coconut, shredded	2 Tbsp
Coffee whitener, liquid	2 Tbsp
Coffee whitener, powdered	4 tsp
Cream (light, coffee, table, sour)	2 Tbsp
Cream (heavy, whipping)	1 Tbsp
Cream cheese	1 Tbsp

Daily Menu Guide/1200 Calories

7 Free Foods

Each free food or drink contains fewer than 20 calories per serving. You may eat as much as you want of free foods that have no portion size given; you may eat two or three servings per day of free foods that have portions listed. Be sure to spread your servings throughout the day.

Drinks

Bouillon or broth, no fat
Cocoa powder, unsweetened baking type (1 Tbsp)
Coffee or tea
Soft drinks, calorie-free, including carbonated drinks

Fruits

Cranberries or rhubarb, no sugar (½ cup)

Sweet Substitutes

Gelatin, sugar-free
Jam or jelly, sugar-free (2 tsp)
Whipped topping (2 Tbsp)

Vegetables (raw, 1 cup)

Cabbage
Celery
Cucumber
Green onion
Hot peppers
Mushrooms
Radishes
Salad greens (as desired):
  Lettuce
  Romaine
  Spinach (raw)
Zucchini

Seasonings can be used as desired. If you are following a low-sodium diet, be sure to read the labels, and choose seasonings that do not contain sodium or salt.

Condiments

Catsup (1 Tbsp)
Dill pickles unsweetened
Horseradish
Hot sauce
Mustard
Salad dressing, low-calorie, including mayonnaise-type (2 Tbsp)
Taco sauce (1 Tbsp)
Vinegar

Flavoring extracts (vanilla, almond, butter, etc.)
Garlic or garlic powder
Herbs, fresh or dried
Lemon or lemon juice
Lime or lime juice

*High in cholesterol.
†Count as 1 meat exchange and 1 fat exchange.

Onion powder
Paprika
Pepper
Pimento
Spices
Soy sauce
Worcestershire sauce

Adapted from Eli Lilly and Company, Indianapolis, Indiana 46286.

297

Daily Menu Guide/1500 Calories
(approximately)

Carbohydrate: 195 gm
Protein: 75 gm
Fat: 50 gm

Breakfast	**Breakfast**
2 Fruit exchanges (List 3)	Orange juice .... 1 cup
2 Bread exchanges (List 4)	Cereal, dry .... ¾ cup
	Toast .... EXAMPLE ...... 1 slice
1 Meat exchange (List 5)	Egg .... EXAMPLE 1
1 Fat exchange (List 6)	Margarine .... 1 tsp
1 cup skim milk (List 1)	Skim milk .... 1 cup
Lunch	**Lunch**
2 Meat exchanges (List 5)	Cold cuts .... 1½-oz. slice
	Cheese .... 1 oz.
2 Bread exchanges (List 4)	Bread .... EXAMPLE ..... 2 slices.
1 Vegetable exchange (List 2)	Carrot and celery sticks .... EXAMPLE ..... ½ cup
2 Fruit exchanges (List 3)	Apples .... 2 small
2 Fat exchanges (List 6)	Mayonnaise-type dressing .... 4 tsp
Dinner	**Dinner**
3 Meat exchanges (List 5)	Chicken, baked .... 3 oz
2 Bread exchanges (List 4)	Peas .... ½ cup
	Potatoes, mashed .... ½ cup
2 Vegetable exchanges (List 2)	Tomatoes .... EXAMPLE .... 1 cup
Vegetable(s) as desired (List 2*)	Lettuce, etc. .... (as desired)
1 Fruit exchange (List 3)	Fruit cocktail .... ½ cup
1 Fat exchange (List 6)	Margarine .... 1 tsp
½ cup skim milk (List 1)	Skim milk.. ½ cup
	French dressing, low-calorie .... 1 Tbsp
Bedtime Snack	**Bedtime Snack**
1 Bread exchange (List 4)	Graham crackers................ EXAMPLE .... 2 squares
½ Cup skim milk (List 1)	Skim milk................................. EXAMPLE .... ½ cup

Daily Menu Guide 1500 Calories (approximately)

Foods Allowed in Reasonable Amounts

Seasonings: Celery salt, cinnamon, garlic, garlic or onion salt, horseradish, lemon, mint, mustard, nutmeg, parsley, pepper, noncaloric sweeteners, spices, vanilla, and vinegar.

Other Foods: Coffee or tea (no sugar or cream), diet beverage without sugar, fat-free broth, bouillon, unflavored gelatin, artificially sweetened fruit-flavored gelatin, sour or dill pickles, and cranberries or rhubarb (without sugar).

List 1 Milk Values

Each portion supplies approximately 12 gm of carbohydrate and 8 gm of protein; the fat content and total calories vary with the type of milk. (One fat exchange equals 5 gm of fat.)

	measurement	fat exchanges	calories
Milk			
Buttermilk	1 cup	—	80
Evaporated, undiluted			
Skim	½ cup	—	80
Whole	½ cup	2	170
Nonfat dry milk mixed according to directions on box	1 cup	—	80
Nonfat dry milk powder	⅓ cup	—	80
Skim	1 cup	—	80
1% butterfat	1 cup	½	107
2% butterfat	1 cup	1	125
Whole	1 cup	2	170
Yogurt, plain made with skim milk	1 cup	—	80

If substitution for the milk indicated in the diet plan is desired, choose either a milk product that contains the same number of fat exchanges or allow for the difference in the meal plan. For example, if the diet plan calls for 1 cup of skim milk (no fat exchange), substitute 1 cup of 2% milk by omitting one fat exchange.

List 2 Vegetable Exchanges

Each portion (except for vegetables marked with an *) supplies approximately 5 gm of carbohydrate and 2 gm of protein, or 25 calories. One serving equals ½ cup.

Asparagus
Beans, green or yellow
Bean sprouts
Beets
Broccoli
Brussels sprouts
Cabbage
Carrots
Cauliflower
Celery
*Chicory
*Chinese cabbage
Cucumbers
Eggplant
*Endive
*Escarole
Greens: beet, chard, collard, dandelion, kale, mustard, spinach, turnip
*Lettuce
Mushrooms
Okra
Onions
*Parsley
Peppers, green or red
*Radishes
Rutabagas
Sauerkraut
Squash, summer
Tomatoes
Tomato juice
Turnips
Vegetable juice cocktail
*Watercress
Zucchini

*May be used as desired.

List 3 Fruit Exchanges

(fresh, dried, frozen, or canned without sugar or syrup)

Each portion supplies approximately 10 gm of carbohydrates, or 4 calories.

	measurement
Apple	1 small (2 in. diam.)
Apple juice or cider	1 cup
Applesauce	½ cup
Apricots, fresh	2 med.
Apricots, dried	4 halves
Banana	½ small
Berries (boysenberries, blackberries, blueberries, raspberries)	½ cup
Cantaloupe	¼ (6-in. diam.)
Cherries	10 large
Dates	2
Figs, fresh	1 large
Figs, dried	1 small
Fruit cocktail	½ cup
Grapefruit	½ small
Grapefruit juice	½ cup
Grapes	12
Grape juice	¼ cup
Honeydew melon	⅛ (7-in. diam.)
Mandarin oranges	¾ cup
Mango	½ small
Nectarine	1 small
Orange	1 small
Orange juice	½ cup
Papaya	¾ cup
Peach	1 med.
Pear	1 small
Persimmon, native	1 med.
Pineapple	½ cup
Pineapple juice	a cup
Plums	2 med.
Prunes	2 med.
Prune juice	¼ cup
Raisins	2 Tbsp
Strawberries	¾ cup
Tangerine	1 large
Watermelon	1 cup

List 4 Bread Exchanges

Each portion supplies approximately 15 gm of carbohydrate and 2 gm of protein, or 70 calories.

	measurement
Bread, French, raisin (without icing), rye, white, whole-wheat	1 slice
Bagel	½
Biscuit, roll	1 (2 in. diam.)
Bread crumbs, dried	3 Tbsp
Bun (for hamburger or wiener)	½

Daily Menu Guide 1500 Calories (approximately)

Cornbread	1 in. × 2 in. × 2 in.
English muffin	½
Muffin	1 (2-in. diam.)
1/20 Cake, angel or sponge, without icing	1½-in. cube (of 10-in.–diam.cake)
Cereal, cooked	½ cup
Dry (flaked or puffed)	¾ cup
Cornstarch	2 Tbsp
Crackers, graham	2 (2½-in. sq)
Oyster	20 (½ cup)
Round	6
Rye wafer	3 (2 in. × 3½ in.)
Saltine	6
Variety	5 small
Flour	2½ Tbsp
Matzoth	1 (6-in. diam.)
Popcorn, popped, unbuttered, small-kernel	1½ cups
Pretzels (3-ring)	6
Rice or grits, cooked	½ cup
Spaghetti, macaroni, noodles, cooked	½ cup
Tortilla	1 (6-in. diam.)
Vegetables	
Beans, baked, without pork	¼ cup
Lima, navy, etc., dry, cooked	½ cup
Corn	1 cup
Corn on the cob	½ med. ear
Parsnips	1 cup
Peas, dried (split peas, etc.) or green, cooked	½ cup
Potatoes, sweet, or yams, fresh	¼ cup
White, baked or boiled	1 (2-in. diam.)
White, mashed	½ cup
Pumpkin	¾ cup
Squash, winter (acorn or butternut)	½ cup
Wheat germ	¼ cup

List 5 Meat Exchanges

Each portion supplies approximately 7 gm of protein and 5 gm of fat, or 73 calories.

	measurement
Cheese, cheddar, American, Swiss	1-oz slice (3½-in. sq, ⅛-in. thick)
Cottage	¼ cup
Egg	1
Fish and seafood	
Halibut, perch, sole, etc.	1-oz slice (4 in. × 2 in. × ¼ in.)
Oysters, clams, shrimp, scallops	5 small
Salmon, tuna, crab	¼ cup
Sardines	3 med.
Meat and poultry	
Beef, lamb, pork, veal, ham, liver, chicken, etc. (med. fat)	1-oz. slice (4 in. × 2 in. × ¼ in.)
Cold cuts	1½-oz. slice (4½-in. sq, ⅛-in. thick)
Vienna sausages	2
† Wiener	1 (10 per lb)
Peanut butter (omit two additional fat exchanges)	2 Tbsp

†Limit wieners to one exchange per day.

List 6 Fat Exchanges

Each portion supplies approximately 5 gm of fat, or 45 calories.

	measurement
Avocado	⅛ (4-in. diam.)
Bacon, crisp	1 slice
Butter or margarine	1 tsp
Cream, half-and-half	3 Tbsp
Heavy, 40%	1 Tbsp
Light, 20%	2 Tbsp
Sour	2 Tbsp
Cream cheese	1 Tbsp
Dressing, French	1 Tbsp
Italian	1 Tbsp
Mayonnaise	1 tsp
Mayonnaise-type	2 tsp
Roquefort	2 tsp
Nuts	6 small
Oil or cooking fat	1 tsp
Olives	5 small

Miscellaneous Foods

The following foods may be used, if you wish, but they must be figured into the daily diet plan, with the food exchanges allowed as indicated.

	measurement	exchanges
Fish sticks, frozen	3 sticks	1 bread, 2 meat
Fruit-flavored gelatin	¼ cup	1 bread
Ginger ale	7 oz.	1 bread
Ice cream, vanilla, chocolate, strawberry	½ cup	1 bread, 2 fat
Low-calorie dressing, French or Italian	1 Tbsp	— ‡
Potato or corn chips	10 larger or 15 small	1 bread, 2 fat
Sherbet	½ cup	2 bread
Vanilla wafers	6	1 bread
Waffle, frozen	1 (5½ in.)	1 bread, 1 fat

‡The fat and calorie contents do not have to be counted if the amount is limited to 1 tablespoonful.

Adapted from Eli Lilly and Company, Indianapolis, Indiana 46286.

Carbohydrate: 349 gm
Protein: 97 gm
Fat: 76 gm

Daily Menu Guide/2500 Calories

Breakfast
2 Fruit (List 4) — 1 cup orange juice
3 Starch/bread (List 1) — ¾ cup ready-to-eat cereal, 2 slices whole wheat toast
Fat (List 6) — 2 tsp margarine
1 Milk (List 5) — 1 cup 1% milk
*Free foods (List 7) — Coffee or tea

Lunch
2 Meat (List 2) — ½ cup tuna
4 Starch/bread (List 1) — 4 slices rye bread
1 Vegetable (List 3) — 1 large tomato
1 Fruit (List 4) — ½ banana
2 Fat (List 6) — 4 tsp salad dressing, mayonnaise- type
*Free foods (List 7) — ½ cup chopped celery

Afternoon Snack
1 Fruit (List 4) — 1 small apple
2 Starch/bread (List 1) — 1½ oz. pretzels

Dinner
3 Meat (List 2) — 3 oz. roast beef
3 Starch/bread (List 1) — 1 small potato, ½ cup corn, 1 slice whole wheat bread
1 Vegetable (List 3) — ½ cup broccoli
2 Fruit (List 4) — 1¼ cup strawberries, a cup grape juice
2 Fat (List 6) — 2 tsp margarine
*Free foods (List 7) — Salad greens, radishes, 2 Tbsp low-calorie salad dressing

Evening Snack
2 Starch/bread (List 1) — 6 Graham crackers
1 Milk (List 5) — 1 cup 1% milk
1 Fruit (List 4) — 1 cup canned pineapple
1 Fat (List 6) — 1 Tbsp cream cheese

*Choose no more than three portions daily of those items that have a serving size given on the Free Food list.

1 Starches and Breads

One portion of each food in this list contains about 15 gm carbohydrate, 3 gm protein, a trace of fat, and 80 calories.
To choose a similar portion of a starch or bread not listed, follow these general rules:
• Cereal, grain, pasta—½ cup
• Bread product—1 oz

Breads

Breads	Portion
Bagel	½ (1 oz.)
Bun (hamburger, hot dog)	½ (1 oz.)
English muffin	½
Pita (6 in. across)	½
Tortilla, flour or corn (6 in. across)	1
Whole wheat, rye, white, pumpernickel, raisin (no icing)	1 slice (1 oz.)

Cereals/Grains/Pasta

Bran cereal, concentrated, such as Bran Buds, All-Bran	⅓ cup
Bran cereal, flaked	½ cup
Cooked cereal, grits, bulgur	½ cup
Grapenuts	3 Tbsp
Macaroni, noodles, spaghetti (cooked)	½ cup
Puffed cereal	1½ cup
Ready-to-eat cereal, unsweetened	¾ cup
Rice, white or brown	⅓ cup
Shredded wheat	½ cup
Wheat germ	3 Tbsp

Crackers/Snacks

Graham cracker (2½ in. square)	3
Matzo	¾ oz.
Melba toast	5 slices

Daily Menu Guide/2500 Calories

Oyster crackers	24
Popcorn, popped, no fat added	3 cups
Pretzels	¾ oz.
Ry Krisp (2 in. × 3½ in.)	4

Starchy Vegetables

Beans, baked	¼ cup
Corn	½ cup or 6-in. cob
Lentils, beans, or peas (dried), such as kidney, white, split, black-eyed	1 cup
Lima beans	½ cup
Peas, green (canned or frozen)	½ cup
Potato, baked	1 small (3 oz.)
Potato, mashed	½ cup
Winter squash (acorn, butternut)	¾ cup
Yam or sweet potato, plain	1 cup

Starch Foods Prepared with Fat

(Count as 1 starch/bread exchange and 1 fat exchange)

Biscuit (2½ in. across)	1
Chow mein noodles	½ cup
Corn bread (2-in. cube)	1 (2 oz.)
Cracker, round butter type	6
French fried potatoes (2–3½ in. long)	10 (1½ oz.)
Muffin (small, plain)	1
Taco shell (6 in. across)	2

2 Meats and Meat Substitutes

One portion of each food in this list contains about 7 gm protein. Lean meats and meat substitutes have about 55 calories per serving; other meat items have 78 to 100 calories per serving. To follow a diet low in cholesterol and saturated fat, choose the lean meats, fish, and other items that appear in bold type. Portions are weighed after cooking and with skin, bones, and fat removed.

	Portion
Beef	
Lean cuts, such as USDA Good/Choice round, sirloin, or flank steak, tenderloin, chipped beef	1 oz.
All other cuts	1 oz.
Cheese	
Cottage or ricotta	¼ cup
Diet (less than 55 calories per oz.)	1 oz.
Parmesan, grated	2 Tbsp
Other cheese (except cream cheese)	1 oz.
Eggs	
Egg substitute (less than 55 calories per ¼ cup)	¼ cup
Egg white	3
Egg, whole*	1
Fish and Seafood	
All fresh or frozen fish	1 oz.
Clams, crab, lobster, shrimp, scallops	2 oz.
Herring, smoked	1 oz.
Oysters	6 medium
Sardines (canned)	2 medium
Tuna (water-packed)	¼ cup
Salmon (canned)	¼ cup
Miscellaneous	
Hot dog† (10 per lb)	1
Lamb (all cuts)	1 oz.
Liver,* heart,* kidney,* sweet breads*	1 oz.
Luncheon meats—**95% fat free;** all others	1 oz.
Peanut butter	1 Tbsp
Sausages, such as Polish, Italian, smoked	1 oz.
Pork	
Lean cuts, such as Canadian bacon; fresh ham; canned, cured, boiled ham; tenderloin	1 oz.
Other cuts	1 oz.

Poultry

Chicken, turkey, Cornish hen (skin removed)	1 oz.

Veal

Lean chops and roasts	1 oz.
Cutlets	1 oz.

3 Vegetables

One portion of each vegetable in this list contains about 5 gm carbohydrate, 2 gm protein, and 25 calories. If no portion size is listed, the following measurements should be used:

• Cooked vegetables or juice—½ cup
• Raw vegetables—1 cup

Check Free Foods (List 7) and Starches/Breads (List 1) for vegetables not listed here.

Asparagus
Beans (green, wax, Italian)
Bean sprouts
Beets
Broccoli
Brussels sprouts
Cabbage (cooked)
Carrots
Cauliflower
Eggplant
Greens (collard, mustard, etc.)
Mushrooms (cooked)
Okra
Onion
Peapods (snow peas)
Peppers (green)
Sauerkraut
Spinach (cooked)
Summer squash (crookneck)
Tomato (1 large)
Tomato or vegetable juice
Turnip
Water chestnuts
Zucchini (cooked)

4 Fruits

One portion of each fruit here contains about 15 gm carbohydrate and 60 calories. To choose a similar portion of a fruit not listed, follow these general rules:

Daily Menu Guide/2500 Calories

- Fresh, canned, or frozen fruit, no sugar added—½ cup
- Dried fruit—¼

	Portion
Apple, raw (2 in. across)	1
Applesauce, no sugar added	½ cup
Apricot, raw (medium)	4
Banana (9 in. long)	½
Blackberries or blueberries, raw	¼ cup
Cantaloupe or honeydew melon	1 cup
Cherries, raw (large)	12
Fig, raw (2 in. across)	2
Fruit cocktail, canned	½ cup
Grapefruit segments	¾ cup
Grapes (small)	15
Kiwi (large)	1
Mandarin orange	¾ cup
Nectarine (2½ in. across)	1
Orange (2½ in. across)	1
Papaya	1 cup
Peach (2¾ in. across)	1 whole or ¾ cup
Pear	½ large or 1 small
Persimmon (native, medium)	2
Pineapple, fresh	¾ cup
Pineapple, canned	⅓ cup
Plum, raw (2 in. across)	2
Raspberries, raw	1 cup
Strawberries, raw (whole)	1¼ cup
Tangerine (2½ in. across)	2
Watermelon	1¼ cup

Dried Fruits

Apple	4 rings
Apricot	7 halves
Date (medium)	2½
Fig	1½
Prune (medium)	3
Raisins	2 Tbsp

Fruit Juices

Apple juice or cider	½ cup
Cranberry juice cocktail	1 cup
Grape juice	1 cup
Prune juice	1 cup
Other, such as orange, pineapple, etc.	½ cup

5 Milk and Milk Products

One portion of each milk or milk product on this list contains about 12 gm carbohydrate and 8 gm protein. These foods also contain 1 to 8 gm fat and 90 to 150 calories per serving, depending on their butterfat content. Choose foods from the skim and lowfat milk groups as often as possible, because they contain less butterfat than do whole milk products.

Skim and Very Lowfat Milk

Skim, ½%, or 1% milk	1 cup
Buttermilk, lowfat	1 cup
Evaporated skim milk	½ cup
Nonfat dry milk	1 cup
Nonfat yogurt, plain	8 oz.

Lowfat Milk
(Count as 1 milk exchange and 1 fat exchange)

2% milk	1 cup
Lowfat yogurt, plain (with added nonfat milk solids)	8 oz.

Whole Milk
(Count as 1 milk exchange and 2 fat exchanges)

Whole milk	1 cup
Evaporated whole milk	½ cup
Whole yogurt, plain	8 oz.

6 Fats

One portion of each food on this list contains about 5 gm fat and 45 calories. Choose unsaturated fats instead of saturated fats as often as possible.

Unsaturated Fats	Portion
Almonds, dry roasted	6 whole
Avocado (medium)	⅛
Margarine	1 tsp
Margarine, diet	1 Tbsp
Mayonnaise	1 tsp
Oil (corn, cottonseed, olive, peanut, safflower, soybean, sunflower)	1 tsp
Olives	10 small or 5 large
Peanuts	20 small or 10 large
Pecans or walnuts	2 whole
Salad dressing, mayonnaise-type	2 tsp
Salad dressing, other varieties	1 Tbsp
Sunflower seeds	1 Tbsp

Saturated Fats	
Bacon	1 slice
Butter	1 tsp
Coconut, shredded	2 Tbsp
Coffee whitener, liquid	2 Tbsp
Coffee whitener, powdered	4 tsp
Cream (light, coffee, table, sour)	2 Tbsp
Cream (heavy, whipping)	1 Tbsp
Cream cheese	1 Tbsp

7 Free Foods

Each free food or drink contains fewer than 20 calories per serving. You may eat as much as you want of free foods that have no portion size given; you may eat two or three servings per day of free foods that have portions listed. Be sure to spread your servings throughout the day.

Drinks

Bouillon or broth, no fat
Cocoa powder, unsweetened baking type (1 Tbsp)
Coffee or tea
Soft drinks, calorie-free, including carbonated drinks

Fruits

Cranberries or rhubarb, no sugar (½ cup)

Sweet substitutes

Gelatin, sugar-free
Jam or jelly, sugar-free (2 tsp)
Whipped topping (2 Tbsp)

Vegetables (raw, 1 cup)

Cabbage
Celery
Cucumber
Green onion
Hot peppers
Mushrooms
Radishes
Salad greens (as desired):
  Lettuce
  Romaine
  Spinach (raw)
Zucchini

Condiments

Catsup (1 Tbsp)
Dill pickles unsweetened
Horseradish
Hot sauce
Mustard
Salad dressing, low-calorie, including mayonnaise-type (2 Tbsp)
Taco sauce (1 Tbsp)
Vinegar

Seasonings can be used as desired. If you are following a low-sodium diet, be sure to read the labels and choose seasonings that do not contain sodium or salt.

Flavoring extracts (vanilla, almond, butter, etc.)
Garlic or garlic powder
Herbs, fresh or dried
Lemon or lemon juice
Lime or lime juice
Onion powder
Paprika
Pepper
Pimento
Spices
Soy sauce
Worcestershire sauce

*High in cholesterol.
†Count as 1 meat exchange and 1 fat exchange.

Adapted from Eli Lilly and Company, Indianapolis, Indiana 46286.

Daily Menu Guide/3000 Calories (approximately)

Carbohydrate: 375 gm
Protein: 150 gm
Fat: 100 gm

Breakfast	**Breakfast**
2 Fruit exchanges (List 3)	Orange juice ....1 cup
3 Bread exchanges (List 4)	Cereal, dry..¾ cup
	Toast ....2 slices
1 Meat exchange (List 5)	Egg 1
2 Fat exchanges (List 6)	Margarine ....2 tsp
1 cup skim milk (List 1)	Skim milk ....1 cup
Midmorning Feeding	**Midmorning Feeding**
1½ Bread exchanges (List 4)	Graham crackers....................................3 squares
½ cup skim milk (List 1)	Skim milk ....½ cup
Lunch	**Lunch**
3 Meat exchanges (List 5)	Cheese ....1 oz. ⎫
4 Bread exchanges (List 4)	Bread..2 slices ⎬ sandwich
3 Fat exchanges (List 6)	Mayonnaise-type dressing......................2 tsp ⎭
	Cold cuts.....................2 1½-oz. slices ⎫
	Bread..2 slices ⎬ sandwich
	Margarine ....2 tsp ⎭
2 Vegetable exchanges (List 2)	Carrots and celery sticks..........................1 cup
2 Fruit exchanges (List 3)	Apples...2 small
1 cup skim milk (List 1)	Skim milk ....1 cup
Midafternoon Feeding	**Midafternoon Feeding**
1 Meat exchange (List 5)	Wiener 1
2 Bread exchanges (List 4)	Wiener bun 1
1 Fruit exchange (List 3)	Grapefruit juice ....½ cup
	Mustard ....as desired
Dinner	**Dinner**
4 Meat exchanges (List 5)	Chicken, baked ....4 oz.
4 Bread exchanges (List 4)	Peas...½ cup
	Potatoes, mashed..½ cup
	Bread ....2 slices
2 Vegetable exchanges (List 2)	Tomatoes ....1 cup
Vegetable(s) as desired (List 2*)	Lettuce, etc. ....as desired
1 Fruit exchange (List 3)	Fruit cocktail ....½ cup
3 Fat exchanges (List 6)	Margarine ....3 tsp
1 cup skim milk (List 1)	Skim milk ....1 cup
Bedtime Feeding	**Bedtime Feeding**
2 Meat exchanges (List 5)	Roast beef, lean.......................................2 oz
2 Bread exchanges (List 4)	Hamburger bun...1
1 Fat exchange (List 6)	Mayonnaise-type dressing ....2 tsp
½ cup skim milk (List 1)	Skim milk ....½ cup

Daily Menu Guide/3000 Calories (approximately)

Foods Allowed in Reasonable Amounts

Seasonings: Celery salt, cinnamon, garlic, garlic or onion salt, horseradish, lemon, mint, mustard, nutmeg, parsley, pepper, noncaloric sweeteners, spices, vanilla, and vinegar.

Other Foods: Coffee or tea (no sugar or cream), diet beverage without sugar, fat-free broth, bouillon, unflavored gelatin, artificially sweetened fruit-flavored gelatin, sour or dill pickles, and cranberries or rhubarb (without sugar).

List 1 Milk Values

Each portion supplies approximately 12 gm of carbohydrate and 8 gm of protein; the fat content and total calories vary with the type of milk.
(One fat exchange equals 5 gm of fat.)

	measurement	fat exchanges	calories
Milk			
Buttermilk	1 cup	—	80
Evaporated, undiluted			
Skim	½ cup	—	80
Whole	½ cup	2	170
Nonfat dry milk mixed according to directions on box	1 cup	—	80
Nonfat dry milk powder	1 cup	—	80
Skim	1 cup	—	80
1% butterfat	1 cup	½	107
2% butterfat	1 cup	1	125
Whole	1 cup	2	170
Yogurt, plain, made with skim milk	1 cup	—	80

If substitution for the milk indicated in the diet plan is desired, choose either a milk product that contains the same number of fat exchanges or allow for the difference in the meal plan. For example, if the diet plan calls for 1 cup of skim milk (no fat exchange), substitute 1 cup of 2% milk by omitting one fat exchange.

List 2 Vegetable Exchanges

Each portion (except for vegetables marked with an *) supplies approximately 5 gm of carbohydrate and 2 gm of protein, or 25 calories. One serving equals ½ cup.

Asparagus
Beans, green or yellow
Bean sprouts
Beets
Broccoli
Brussels sprouts
Cabbage
Carrots
Cauliflower
Celery
*Chicory
*Chinese cabbage
Cucumbers
Eggplant
*Endive
*Escarole
Greens: beet, chard, collard, dandelion, kale, mustard, spinach, turnip
*Lettuce
Mushrooms
Okra
Onions
*Parsley
Peppers, green or red
*Radishes
Rutabagas
Sauerkraut
Squash, summer
Tomatoes
Tomato juice
Turnips
Vegetable juice cocktail
*Watercress
Zucchini

*May be used as desired.

List 3 Fruit Exchanges

(fresh, dried, frozen, or canned without sugar or syrup)
Each portion supplies approximately 10 gm of carbohydrates, or 40 calories.

	measurement
Apple	1 small (2-in. diam.)
Apple juice or cider	1 cup
Applesauce	½ cup
Apricots, fresh	2 med.
Apricots, dried	4 halves
Banana	½ small
Berries (boysenberries, blackberries, blueberries, raspberries)	½ cup
Cantaloupe	¼ (6-in. diam.)
Cherries	10 large
Dates	2
Figs, fresh	1 large
Figs, dried	1 small
Fruit cocktail	½ cup
Grapefruit	½ small
Grapefruit juice	½ cup
Grapes	12
Grape juice	¼ cup
Honeydew melon	⅛ (7-in. diam.)
Mandarin oranges	¾ cup
Mango	½ small
Nectarine	1 small
Orange	1 small
Orange juice	½ cup
Papaya	¾ cup
Peach	1 med.
Pear	1 small
Persimmon, native	1 med.
Pineapple	½ cup
Pineapple juice	1 cup
Plums	2 med.
Prunes	2 med.
Prune juice	¼ cup
Raisins	2 Tbsp
Strawberries	¾ cup
Tangerine	1 large
Watermelon	1 cup

List 4 Bread Exchanges

Each portion supplies approximately 15 gm of carbohydrate and 2 gm of protein, or 70 calories.

	measurement
Bread, French, raisin (without icing), rye, white, whole-wheat	1 slice
Bagel	½

Daily Menu Guide/3000 Calories (approximately)

Biscuit, roll	1 (2-in. diam.)
Bread crumbs, dried	3 Tbsp
Bun (for hamburger or wiener)	1/2
Cornbread	1 in. × 2 in. × 2 in.
English muffin	1/2
Muffin	1 (2-in. diam.)
Cake, angel or sponge, without icing	1 1/2 in. cube (1/20 of 10-in.–diam.cake)
Cereal, cooked	1/2 cup
Dry (flaked or puffed)	3/4 cup
Cornstarch	2 Tbsp
Crackers, graham	2 (2 1/2-in. sq)
Oyster	20 (1/2 cup)
Round	6
Rye wafer	3 (2 in. × 3 1/2 in.)
Saltine	6
Variety	5 small
Flour	2 1/2 Tbsp
Matzoth	1 (6 in. diam.)
Popcorn, popped, unbuttered, small-kernel	1 1/2 cups
Pretzels (3-ring)	6
Rice or grits, cooked	1/2 cup
Spaghetti, macaroni, noodles, cooked	1/2 cup
Tortilla	1 (6 in. diam.)
Vegetables	
Beans, baked, without pork	1/4 cup
Lima, navy, etc. dry, cooked	1/2 cup
Corn	1/3 cup
Corn on the cob	1/2 med. ear
Parsnips	2/3 cup
Peas, dried (split peas, etc.) or green, cooked	1/2 cup
Potatoes, sweet or yams, fresh	1/4 cup
White, baked or boiled	1 (2-in. diam.)
White, mashed	1/2 cup
Pumpkin	3/4 cup
Squash, winter (acorn or butternut)	1/2 cup
Wheat germ	1/4 cup

List 5 Meat Exchanges

Each portion supplies approximately 7 gm of protein and 5 gm of fat, or 73 calories.

	measurement
Cheese, cheddar, American, Swiss	1-oz. slice (3 1/2-in. sq, 1/8-in. thick)
Cottage	1/4 cup
Egg	1
Fish and seafood	
Halibut, perch, sole, etc.	1-oz. slice (4 in. × 2 in. × 1/4 in.)
Oysters, clams, shrimp, scallops	5 small
Salmon, tuna, crab	1/4 cup
Sardines	3 med.
Meat and poultry	
Beef, lamb, pork, veal, ham, liver, chicken, etc. (med. fat)	1-oz. slice (4 in. × 2 in. × 1/4 in.)
Cold cuts	1 1/2-oz. slice (4 1/2-in. sq, 1/8-in. thick)
Vienna sausages	2
†Wiener	1 (10 per lb)
Peanut butter (omit two additional fat exchanges)	2 Tbsp

†Limit wieners to one exchange per day.

List 6 Fat Exchanges

Each portion supplies approximately 5 gm of fat, or 45 calories.

	measurement
Avocado	1/8 (4-in. diam.)
Bacon, crisp	1 slice
Butter or margarine	1 tsp
Cream, half-and-half	3 Tbsp
Heavy, 40%	1 Tbsp
Light, 20%	2 Tbsp
Sour	2 Tbsp
Cream cheese	1 Tbsp
Dressing, French	1 Tbsp
Italian	1 Tbsp
Mayonnaise	1 tsp
Mayonnaise-type	2 tsp
Roquefort	2 tsp
Nuts	6 small
Oil or cooking fat	1 tsp
Olives	5 small

Miscellaneous foods

The following foods may be used, if you wish, but they must be figured into the daily diet plan, with the food exchanges allowed as indicated.

	measurement	exchange
Fish sticks, frozen	3 sticks	1 bread, 2 meat
Fruit-flavored gelatin	1/4 cup	1 bread
Ginger ale	7 oz.	1 bread
Ice cream, vanilla, chocolate, strawberry	1/2 cup	1 bread, 2 fat
Low-calorie dressing, French or Italian	1 Tbsp	—‡
Potato or corn chips	10 larger or 15 small	1 bread, 2 fat
Sherbet	1/2 cup	2 bread
Vanilla wafers	6	1 bread
Waffle, frozen	1 (5 1/2 in.)	1 bread,1 fat

‡ The fat and calorie contents do not have to be counted if the amount is limited to 1 tablespoonful.

Adapted from Eli Lilly and Company, Indianapolis, Indiana 46286.

PURPOSE

This diet is often used to minimize digestion within the gastrointestinal tract. Fluid and energy are provided in a form to minimize digestion.

DESCRIPTION

The diet consists of clear liquids or foods that are fluid at body temperature.

BASIC INFORMATION

Due to the extremely restrictive nature of this diet, use should be limited to 3 days or less. For prolonged use, an appropriate low-residue supplement is recommended for nutritional support.

NUTRITIONAL ADEQUACY

This diet is extremely inadequate and is planned for brief use only. Specific items and amounts depend upon patient tolerance and should be offered frequently.

FOOD LISTS

Food Groups	Foods Allowed	Foods to Omit
Milk/Dairy	None	All
Meat Substitutes	None	All
Breads/Grains	None	All
Fruits/Vegetables	Clear fruit juices, such as: apple, grape, or cranberry, or strained juices, such as orange, lemonade or grapefruit, lemonade, pulp-free fruit ices.	All others
Desserts/Sweets	Clear, flavored gelatin, Popsicles, clear fruit ices, sugar, honey, sugar substitutes, hard candy.	All others
Beverages	Clear coffee or tea, carbonated beverages, sports drinks.	All others, including milk, nectars, cream, juices with pulp.
Miscellaneous	High-protein broth or gelatin, iodized salt, clear broth, or bouillon.	All others

SAMPLE MENU

Breakfast	Dinner or Lunch	Supper or Lunch
Grape Juice	Apple Juice	Cranberry Juice
Clear Broth	Clear Beef Broth	Clear Chicken Broth
Flavored Gelatin	Flavored Gelatin	Flavored Gelatin
Black Coffee	Clear Tea	Clear Tea

Nutrient Analysis

Calories	512 Kcal	Riboflavin	0.3 mg
Protein	19 gm	Thiamin	0.1 mg
Carbohydrate	105 gm	Folate	18 mcg
Fat	4 gm	Calcium	56 mg
Cholesterol	0 mg	Phosphorus	203 mg
Dietary Fiber	0 gm	Zinc	1 mg
Vitamin A	1 RE	Iron	2 mg
Vitamin C	46 mg	Sodium	2346 mg
Niacin	9 mg	Potassium	888 mg

From Griffith HW. Instructions for Patients, 5th ed. Philadelphia, WB Saunders, 1994, p 529. Adapted from Arizona Diet Manual (revised 1992).

PURPOSE

This diet is intended for the patient who cannot chew or swallow solid foods or as a transition from the clear liquid to soft or general diet.

DESCRIPTION

This diet is a modification in the consistency or texture of the normal diet. It contains foods that are liquid or will become liquid at body temperature and are free from mechanical irritants.

BASIC INFORMATION

Milk-based foods make up a large proportion of this diet.

NUTRITIONAL ADEQUACY

This diet may be inadequate in niacin, folacin, and iron. If the diet is used for longer than 2 to 3 weeks, a liquid vitamin/mineral supplement is recommended. Patients with lactose intolerance should use a lactose hydrolyzed milk or use lactose-free products.

FULL LIQUID DIET—FOOD LISTS

Food Groups	Foods Allowed	Foods to Avoid
Milk/Dairy	All milk and milk drinks, such as milkshakes and eggnogs made from commercial mix, yogurt-plain or flavored (no seeds or fruit pieces). All beverages, including high-protein, high-calorie oral supplements.	Cheese, cottage cheese
Meat/Meat Substitutes	Eggnogs, custards.	All others
Breads/Grains	Thin, cooked cereal, such as farina, grits, oatmeal.	All others
Fruit/Vegetables	Vitamin C sources (daily): Strained citrus and tomato juices. Vitamin A sources (alternate days): Strained carrot juice.	All others
Desserts/Sweets	Custards, puddings, plain gelatin, plain ice cream, ice milk, sherbet, sugar, hard candy, honey, popsicle, syrup, frozen yogurt.	All others
Miscellaneous	Butter, margarine, cream, nondairy creamer.	All others

SAMPLE MENU

Suggested Meal Plan	Suggested Foods and Beverages
Breakfast Fruit Juice Cereal Meat/Meat Substitute Milk/Dairy Beverage	 Orange Juice, strained Farina Custard 2% Milk Coffee
Dinner—Noon or Evening Meal Soup Juice Salad Dessert Beverage	 Strained Cream Soup Tomato Juice Lime Gelatin Ice Cream Ginger Ale
Snack Milk/Dairy	 1 Milkshake
Supper—Evening or Noon Meal Soup Juice Dessert Beverage	 Strained Cream Soup Peach Nectar Popsicle Chocolate Milk
Snack Juice Milk/Dairy	 Cranberry Juice Vanilla Pudding, 2% Milk

Nutrient Analysis

Calories	1881 Kcal	Riboflavin	2.7 mg
Protein	60 gm	Thiamin	0.9 mg
Carbohydrate	293 gm	Folate	161 mcg
Fat	56 gm	Calcium	1822 mg
Cholesterol	311 mg	Phosphorus	1572 mg
Dietary Fiber	7 gm	Zinc	7 mg
Vitamin A	931 RE	Iron	5 mg
Vitamin C	133 mg	Sodium	3205 mg
Niacin	5 mg	Potassium	3120 mg

From Griffith HW. Instructions for Patients, 5th ed. Philadelphia, WB Saunders, 1994, pp 530–531. Adapted from Arizona Diet Manual (revised 1992).

PURPOSE

As a progression from the full liquid diet to a general diet. The soft diet can also be used for a postoperative patient who is too ill to tolerate a general diet. The soft diet may also be needed for patients who are too weak or whose dentition is too poor to handle all foods on a general diet.

DESCRIPTION

Food tolerances vary with individuals. Tender foods are used (not ground or pureed) unless the individual needs additional modifications. Most raw fruits and vegetables and coarse breads and cereals are eliminated.

BASIC INFORMATION

Fried foods and highly seasoned foods may cause discomfort in the immobile or postoperative patient.

NUTRITIONAL ADEQUACY

The diet will be adequate if foods from each of the basic food groups are eaten daily.

SOFT DIET—FOOD LISTS

Food Groups	Foods Allowed	Foods to Avoid
Milk/Dairy	Milk and milk drinks, milkshakes, cream cheese, cottage cheese, mild cheeses.	Sharp or highly seasoned cheese.
Meat/Meat Substitutes	Broiled, roasted, baked or stewed tender lean beef, mutton, lamb, veal, chicken, turkey, liver, ham, crisp bacon, white fish, tuna, salmon. Eggs, smooth peanut butter.	All fried meats, fish, or fowl. Rich gravies and sauces. Lunchmeats, sausages, hot dogs. Meats with gristle, chunky peanut butter.
Breads/Grains	Rice, noodles, spaghetti, macaroni. Dry or cooked refined cereals, such as farina, cream of wheat, oatmeal, grits, whole wheat cereals. Plain or toasted white or wheat blend or whole grain breads, soda crackers or saltines, flour tortillas. Broths or creamed soups made with allowed vegetables, strained tomatoes.	Wild rice, coarse cereals, such as bran. Seed in or on breads and crackers. Bread or bread products with nuts or seeds. All others that are not made with allowed vegetables. Highly seasoned soups.
Fruits/Vegetables	Fruit and vegetable juices, well cooked or canned fruits and vegetables, any dried fruit. One citrus fruit daily, one vitamin A source daily. Well ripened, easy to chew fruits, sweet potatoes. Baked, boiled, mashed, creamed, escalloped or au gratin potatoes.	All gas-forming vegetables (corn, radishes, Brussels sprouts, onions, broccoli, cabbage, parsnips, turnips, chili peppers, pinto beans, split peas, dried beans). Fruits containing seeds and skin. Potato chips and corn chips.
Desserts/Sweets	Simple desserts, such as custard, junkets, gelatin desserts, plain ice cream and sherbets, simple cakes and cookies, allowed fruits, sugar, syrup, jelly, honey, plain hard candy, and molasses.	Rich pastries, any dessert containing dates, nuts, raisins, or coconut. Fried pastries, such as doughnuts. Chocolate.
Beverages	Fruit and vegetable juices, caffeine-free carbonated drinks, coffee, and tea.	Caffeinated beverages: coffee, tea, colas.
Miscellaneous	Butter, cream, margarine, mayonnaise, oil. Cream sauces, salt, and mild spices.	Highly spiced salad dressings. Highly seasoned foods, Tabasco, mustard or horseradish, and pepper.

SAMPLE MENU

Suggested Meal Plan	Suggested Foods and Beverages
Breakfast	
Fruit Juice	Orange Juice
Cereal	Oatmeal
Meat/Meat Substitute	Soft Cooked Egg
Bread/Margarine	Toast/Margarine[*]
Milk/Dairy	2% Milk[*]
Beverage	Coffee
Dinner—Noon or Evening Meal	
Meat/Meat Substitute	Meat Loaf
Potato/Potato Substitute	Mashed Potato
Vegetable and/or Salad	Green Beans
Dessert	Lemon Pudding
Bread/Margarine	Bread/Margarine[*]
Beverage	Coffee
Supper—Evening or Noon Meal	
Soup or Juice	Apricot Nectar, Consommé
Meat/Meat Substitute	Chicken Breast
Vegetable and/or Salad	Rice, Peas, and Carrots
Dessert	Applesauce
Bread/Margarine	Bread/Margarine[*]
Milk	2% Milk[*]

[*]To reduce amount of fat in your diet, omit margarine and use 1% or skim milk.

Nutrient Analysis

Calories	1953 Kcal	Riboflavin	2.0 mg
Protein	102 gm	Thiamin	1.5 mg
Carbohydrate	247 gm	Folate	249 mcg
Fat	65 gm	Calcium	1030 mg
Cholesterol	449 mg	Phosphorus	1782 mg
Dietary Fiber	19 gm	Zinc	12 mg
Vitamin A	2944 RE	Iron	13 mg
Vitamin C	79 mg	Sodium	2994 mg
Niacin	25 mg	Potassium	3046 mg

From Griffith HW. Instructions for Patients, 5th ed. Philadelphia, WB Saunders, 1994, pp 542–543. Adapted from Arizona Diet Manual (revised 1992).

Foods Allowed Daily

Foods Allowed Daily	Amount	Protein
Milk	½ cup	4 gm
Eggs	1	7 gm
Meat (lean or meat substitute) (1 oz. cheese, ¼ cup cottage cheese, or ½ cup dried beans equals 1 oz. meat)	2 oz.	14 gm
Potato, rice, macaroni, noodles, etc.	2 servings (½ cup each)	4 gm
Vegetables		
Green leafy or yellow	1 serving (½ cup)	2 gm
Other	1–2	
Fruits and fruit juice	3 servings	
(include 1 citrus serving)	1 cup	
Breads	3 slices	6 gm
Cereals	1 serving (½ cup)	2 gm
Fats, margarine, oil, etc.	As desired	
Cream	¼ cup	1 gm
Sugar, jelly, jam, hard candy	As desired	
Total		40 gm

Note: If salt-free foods are used, the sodium content of this diet is approximately 1 gram.

SAMPLE MENU

Suggested Meal Plan	Sample Menu
Breakfast	
Citrus fruit or juice	Orange juice
½ cup cereal with ½ cup milk	½ cup oatmeal with ½ cup milk
Enriched bread—1 slice—margarine, jelly	1 slice enriched toast, margarine, jelly
1 egg	1 egg
Beverage, cream (¼ cup) and sugar	Coffee/tea, ¼ cup cream, sugar
Dinner (Noon or Evening Meal)	
1 oz. meat or meat substitute	1 oz. serving meat loaf
½ cup potato or potato substitute	½ cup potato
1 vegetable and/or salad	½ cup green beans
	Tossed green salad, oil and vinegar
Fruit	Cantaloupe
1 slice enriched bread—margarine	1 slice enriched bread—margarine
Beverage, sugar	Coffee or tea with sugar
Supper (Evening or Noon Meal)	
1 oz. meat or substitute	1 oz. cheese
½ cup potato or potato substitute	½ cup rice
Vegetable	½ cup peas
Salad	Sliced tomato on lettuce leaf
Fruit	Baked apple, cinnamon
1 slice enriched bread—margarine	1 slice enriched bread—margarine
Beverage, sugar	Coffee or tea, sugar

From Griffith HW. Instructions for Patients, 4th ed. Philadelphia, WB Saunders, 1989, p 108.

BASIC INFORMATION

Potassium is the predominant positively charged electrolyte in body cells. The flow of potassium and sodium in and out of the cells helps maintain the normal functioning of the heart, brain, kidney, and skeletal muscles. It promotes regular heart beat, muscle contractions, and nerve transmissions. A potassium-enriched diet may be recommended for a patient with low serum potassium levels. Low levels of potassium seldom result from dietary deficiency because many foods contain potassium. Instead, the low level is usually due to illness, injury or trauma, or from certain drugs, such as some diuretics and steroids.

Foods High in Potassium	Amount of Serving	Potassium (mg)
Cereals		
Kellogg's All Bran	½ cup	532
Nabisco 100% Bran	½ cup	354
Bran Flakes	1 cup	251
Shredded Wheat	1 cup	155
Fruit		
Orange juice	1 cup	479
Dried apricots	¼ cup	454
Cantaloupe	¼ med.	412
Prunes	¼ cup	353
Banana	1 small	338
Grapefruit juice (canned)	1 cup	360
Tomato juice	1 cup	552
Avocado	½	510
Peaches (dried)	4 med. halves	330
Raisins	3 Tbsp	225
Cooked beans		
Pinto beans	½ cup	531
Kidney beans	½ cup	452
Lentils	½ cup	374
Black beans	½ cup	309
Canned beans	½ cup	332
Vegetables		
Baked potato	1 med.	593
Baked winter squash	1 cup	590
Baked sweet potato	¾ cup	528
Beet greens	½ cup	417
Chard (large leaves)	½ cup	563
Peas (cooked)	½ cup	296
Spinach (fresh)	½ cup	440
Lima beans (canned or frozen)	½ cup	473
Other		
Canned tomato sauce	½ cup	459
Blackstrap molasses	2 Tbsp	1218
Sardines (canned in oil)	3 oz.	459
Chocolate (unsweetened/bitter)	1 oz.	249

According to the Food and Drug Administration's (FDA) food labeling guidelines (effective May 1994), the listing of the potassium content on food products is a voluntary, rather than a mandatory, one. Therefore, even if potassium isn't shown on the label, it can still be a component.

From Griffith HW. Instructions for Patients, 5th ed. Philadelphia, WB Saunders, 1994, p 534.

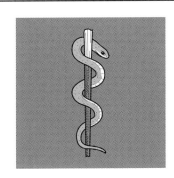
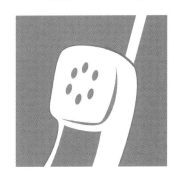

Hematologic Problems

Anemia

Patient and Caregiver's Guide

General Information

Anemia results when the hemoglobin level (red blood cell count) in the blood falls. It is a common problem in elderly patients. Anemia has many possible causes. These include blood loss, destruction of the blood cells by the body, and impaired production of red blood cells. In turn, each of these has its own list of causes. The best treatment for anemia addresses the cause whenever possible. In addition, adequate iron and other blood-forming elements are provided to help speed a return to normal hemoglobin levels.

Anemia causes pallor, fatigue, and weakness. Anemia can worsen the symptoms of other underlying diseases. Anemic patients with angina pectoris (pain from a poor vascular supply to the heart muscle) have chest pain with less exercise or effort. In a patient with heart disease, the strain imposed by anemia may bring on heart failure, marked by ankle swelling and breathlessness. Dizziness and changes in mental status are also possible.

When anemia develops slowly, the body's adjustments may permit normal function, despite very low hemoglobin levels. Because of the patient's gradual adaptation and accommodation to the falling hemoglobin in the blood, symptoms may not appear until the anemia is quite severe. Then, at a certain limit that differs for each patient, symptoms appear in a rush.

Anemia that develops quickly causes symptoms to appear sooner. Although the anemia itself may be a problem, the underlying cause may be a more profound hazard.

Important Points in Treatment

The treatment of simple forms of anemia is oral iron administration. Your physician will determine the cause of the anemia rather than just treat the anemia with replacement iron. The cause may pose far more important health problems than the anemia

319

alone. In addition, treating the cause is important to prevent the recurrence of the anemia after iron therapy is stopped.

Many kinds of anemia necessitate therapy other than with iron. In some unusual cases, iron may even be harmful. Your physician will strive to find the proper combination of treatments to restore your blood count and to prevent any recurrence of the anemia.

Notify Our Office If

- You have unusual pallor or fatigue. Anemia is not so much a disease as it is one result of another disease process. Treatment of the anemia alone, particularly if successful, may result in the oversight of more serious problems. Bring suspicions of anemia to the attention of your physician promptly.

Pernicious Anemia

Patient and Caregiver's Guide ■ ■ ■

General Information

Pernicious anemia occurs when the body lacks vitamin B_{12}. The body requires only a tiny amount of this vitamin, but it is essential. Vitamin B_{12} is found in many foods, but a second substance produced by the stomach is needed for its absorption. This second substance is called *intrinsic factor*. When the lining of the stomach atrophies (wastes away), it no longer makes intrinsic factor. Atrophy of the lining of the stomach is a change that occurs with aging.

The body has vitamin B_{12} in storage. This store can last for years. When this is eventually depleted, anemia begins to develop. Unlike other kinds of anemia, pernicious anemia does not require the loss of blood or a deficiency of iron.

If the anemia progresses for long enough, some changes in the nervous system occur as well. These changes may affect your balance and make it difficult to walk without falling. The other common finding in pernicious anemia is a sore, red tongue.

Important Points in Treatment

Treatment is by injection of vitamin B_{12} or administration by a nasal spray. Once the first month of weekly injections have been completed, it usually takes only one injection per month to prevent the anemia from recurring. Early treatment is necessary to prevent changes in the nervous system, which may not be completely reversible.

Notify Our Office If

- You have a sore, red tongue.
- You experience weakness or difficulty walking.

Vitamin B₁₂ Deficiency

General Information

A deficiency in vitamin B_{12} is a relatively common occurrence in the elderly. This deficiency may occur for a number of different reasons. One form of this deficiency is called *pernicious anemia*. This occurs when changes in the stomach prevent the absorption of the vitamin. Interference with absorption may also be the result of surgery on the stomach or of disease of the small intestine. A few medications also interfere with absorption. It is also possible that with poor nutrition, one may just not get enough vitamin B_{12}.

When this vitamin is not present in adequate amounts, several changes occur in the body. Red blood cells are not properly formed and anemia may develop. With the anemia, one experiences ease of fatigue. Because the stomach may be inflamed, patients may also have symptoms of gastric upset or loss of appetite. Changes in the tongue occur, with the tongue taking on a smooth, almost glossy, appearance. Changes in the nerves occur as well. Patients have difficulty with balance and some loss of sensation, and they may have impairment of memory. A few patients will become depressed or may appear demented.

The diagnosis is readily made with blood tests. On some occasions, tests involving radioactive B_{12} must be done. Diagnosis is important because the changes in the nerves may not be completely reversed by treatment.

Important Points in Therapy

The usual treatment for vitamin B_{12} deficiency is the replacement of the vitamin. In the past, this required monthly injections of the vitamin, but newer forms that may be administered by a nasal spray are now available. If the problem was simple lack of eating enough vitamin B_{12}, oral administration of the drug will be effective. Your physician will guide you in the selection of the form of the vitamin that is best for you.

Notify Our Office If

- You develop difficulty with balance or have an impairment of the ability to recognize objects by touch.
- You develop persistent or recurrent pins-and-needles sensation in your hands or feet.

Multiple Myeloma

Patient and Caregiver's Guide

General Information

Multiple myeloma is a tumor involving blood cells called *plasma cells*. Plasma cell tumors often grow in the bone marrow cavities. The growth of these tumors can cause a replacement of other cells in the bone marrow, with a resultant decrease in the production of other blood cells. Normally, plasma cells produce a protein, a type of antibody, that circulates in the blood. The tumor produces this protein in amounts that can thicken the blood and slow the circulation, which can affect kidney function.

Multiple myeloma usually occurs after age 50 and increases in occurrence with age. Because the tumor grows within bone marrow cavities, bone pain often occurs. The tumor causes a decrease in the production of blood cells, and anemia occurs. Resistance to infection may be impaired, and infections, particularly pneumonia, are frequent.

Important Points in Treatment

Treatment of multiple myeloma is with chemotherapy. Sometimes radiation therapy is used to shrink tumor masses that are causing a problem because of pressure. Drinking extra fluids may help preserve kidney function. Occasionally, removal of serum can reduce the amount of abnormal protein found in the circulation.

Lymphoma

Patient and Caregiver's Guide

General Information

Malignant tumors can occur in any organ system in the body. When the lymph nodes and the lymphatic system are directly involved, the tumor is a lymphoma. Some lymphomas are also called Hodgkin's disease. These tumors may occur at any age, but there is a progressive increase in their occurrence with advancing age.

Often the first sign of lymphoma is the development of a lump. This may be close enough to the skin to be felt, or it may press on an organ and cause symptoms. Usually, your physician needs to obtain some tissue to make the diagnosis and select the proper treatment. Fever, night sweats, weight loss, and itching may also be presenting symptoms.

Important Points in Treatment

There are several varieties of lymphomas. Treatment varies with both the location and the type of lymphoma. Some treatments involve x-ray therapy. Many lymphomas are treated with oral or injected medication. These treatments, called *chemotherapy,* suppress and kill the tumor cells. Some lymphomas are so susceptible to treatment that chemotherapy will cure them. In other cases, there is suppression of the tumor and slowing of its growth. The process of determining the kind and extent of lymphoma is called *staging*. Staging involves a number of x-ray and laboratory examinations and may require surgery.

In Hodgkin's disease, the long-term benefit with treatment is excellent. With other forms of lymphoma, the outcome depends on the type and extent of the tumor. Treatments are in regular courses, and some medications necessitate that frequent visits be made to your physician's office for intravenous injection and tests to monitor the progress of the treatment.

Notify Our Office If

● You notice a lump or feel a mass that was not previously there.

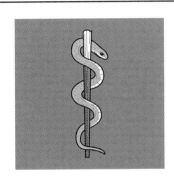
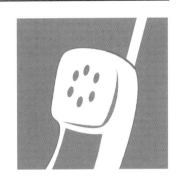

Endocrine Problems

Hypothyroidism

Patient and Caregiver's Guide

General Information

The thyroid is a small gland found in the lower front of the neck. The hormones secreted by the thyroid gland are important for normal metabolism. Disease of the thyroid gland occurs with increased frequency in elderly patients. This increased frequency is largely due to hypothyroidism, or underfunctioning of the thyroid gland. The other major thyroid problem in elderly patients is the development of nodules or lumps in the thyroid gland.

Hypothyroidism is more common in women than in men. It is also more common in people in institutions (such as nursing homes) than in those who remain at home.

Hypothyroidism is most often a result of inflammation of the thyroid gland, called *thyroiditis*. Thyroiditis is a result of abnormal immune reactions by the body against the thyroid gland. Underfunction can also be a result of treatment with radioactive iodine given many years earlier to treat an overactive thyroid gland. Surgical removal of part of the thyroid gland is also a factor in the development of hypothyroidism.

In younger patients, hypothyroidism is manifested by fatigue, dry skin, and constipation. In elderly patients, the signs and symptoms are not so specific. The dry skin, fatigue, and depressive effects occur, but there is also weight loss, decreased appetite, incoordination, confusion, and falls. Many of the signs and symptoms of hypothyroidism in the elderly can be mistakenly attributed to old age. Some elderly patients with hypothyroidism appear to have no symptoms.

Important Points in Treatment

Hypothyroidism is readily treatable. Treatment involves the use of replacement thyroid hormone. The course of treatment is gradual. The hormone is replaced in steps to remain within the tolerance limits of the patient. In elderly patients who may have other

329

health problems, there is limited tolerance for sudden adjustments of thyroid hormone.

Notify Our Office If

- You notice the onset of persistent tiredness or fatigue.
- You notice the development of dry skin or intolerance of cold temperatures.

Thyroid Nodules

Patient and Caregiver's Guide

General Information

Thyroid nodules are tumors, most of which are benign, but some of which are malignant and invasive cancers. These tumors are treatable and increase in frequency with age. They are more common in women. Nodules are an enlargement of the thyroid gland that can often be felt by your physician at the time of a physical examination. In patients with a history of prior radiation treatment to the neck—either near the thyroid gland or near a gland called the *thymus* (such radiation treatment was popular in past decades, although it is no longer used)—the risk of nodules is high. These nodules tend to develop long after the treatment.

In patients who are at high risk but in whom no nodules are felt, other tests are used to identify the presence of nodular change in the thyroid gland. A biopsy of the nodule with a needle may be undertaken, if there is any question of the diagnosis.

Important Points in Treatment

When the diagnosis is a malignant tumor, the treatment is removal of the tumor. For nodules that are not malignant, drug therapy is given, but if the nodules are causing pressure on surrounding tissues, their removal may be in order.

Notify Our Office If

- You note a swelling in your neck. Small lumps, which are enlarged lymph nodes, may come and go with colds, sore throats, or other respiratory infections. Persistent lumps should be brought to the attention of your physician.

Hyperthyroidism

Patient and Caregiver's Guide ▪ ▪ ▪

General Information

When the thyroid gland, a gland in the neck, overfunctions it can secrete thyroid hormone in excess and cause hyperthyroidism. It occurs in elderly patients and is substantially more common in women than in men. In younger patients the excess thyroid hormone causes nervousness, tremor, and weight loss. Patients may appear flushed and warm. Symptoms and signs in the elderly may be much different. Often the excess in thyroid hormone will affect other diseases, particularly heart diseases, causing symptoms or changes to appear without a good explanation. Often the newly emerged symptoms are difficult to treat and control successfully.

In some elderly patients, hyperthyroidism has an unusual, almost reverse presentation, and patients are lethargic rather than hyperactive. These patients develop the problems mentioned previously, with other diseases unexpectedly becoming worse or difficult to treat.

Important Points in Treatment

The usual treatments for hyperthyroidism are medications to reduce the activity of the thyroid gland. These are effective in the elderly. Surgery for removal of the thyroid gland was much used in the past but is not frequently used now.

Notify Our Office If

- You notice an enlargement of the thyroid gland, usually an enlargement in the neck.
- You notice unusual weight loss, nervousness, or sensitivity to heat.
- You become unusually tired, listless, or weak.

Table 14–1 American Urologic Association Symptom Index for Benign Prostatic Hypertrophy

Questions to be asked	Not at all	Less than 1 time in 5	Less than 1/2 the time	About 1/2 the time	More than 1/2 the time	Almost always
			AUA Symptom Score—Circle One Number on Each Line			
1. Over the past month, how often have you had a sensation of not emptying your bladder completely after you finished urination?	0	1	2	3	4	5
2. Over the past month, how often have you had to urinate again, less than 2 hours after you finished urinating?	0	1	2	3	4	5
3. Over the past month, how often have you found that you stopped and started again several times when you urinated?	0	1	2	3	4	5
4. Over the past month, how often have you found it difficult to postpone urination?	0	1	2	3	4	5
5. Over the past month, how often have you had a weak urinary stream?	0	1	2	3	4	5
6. Over the past month, how often have you had to push or strain to begin urination?	0	1	2	3	4	5
7. Over the past month, how many times did you most typically get up to urinate from the time you went to bed at night to the time you got up in the morning?	0 times	1 time	2 times	3 times	4 times	5 times or more

The sum of the 7 circled numbers is the AUA score. _____

A score of 0 to 7 = mild symptoms.
A score of 8 to 19 = moderate symptoms.
A score of 20 to 35 = severe symptoms.
From Barry MJ, Floyd JF Jr, O'Leary MP, et al: The American Urologic Association Symptom Index for benign prostatic hyperplasia. *J Urol* 148:1549–1557, 1992.

Prostatic Cancer

Patient and Caregiver's Guide

General Information

The prostate gland surrounds the urethra, the passageway for urine that leads from the bladder to the outside of the body. Cancer may develop in this gland. Prostatic cancer is a disease of older men. The tumor is often silent and without symptoms, until cancer has spread.

Early symptoms of prostatic cancer are not separable from those of benign prostatic hypertrophy. These symptoms may include:

- *Hesitancy* (difficulty starting the urinary stream)
- *Frequency* (frequent passage of urine)
- *Urgency* (passage of small amounts of urine). Frequently, there is dribbling and a decrease in the force of the urinary stream as well.

As the tumor progresses, it may produce blood in the urine *(hematuria)* or sudden obstruction with urinary retention. Most often the first signs and symptoms may be related to the distant spread of the cancer rather than to problems with the urinary tract itself.

Important Points in Treatment

Prostatic cancer is a slowly progressive tumor. If the physician finds a tumor before it spreads, the treatment is often surgical. Even after spread has occurred, prostatic cancer is only slowly progressive. With radiation and chemotherapy, it is possible to arrest or slow the development of the tumor.

Notify Our Office If

- You note a change in your ability to urinate.
- You see blood in your urine.

Hematuria (Blood in the Urine)

Patient and Caregiver's Guide

General Information

When blood is present in the urine, it is called *hematuria*. If the blood is present in quantities large enough to permit it to be seen, it is called *gross hematuria*. If the blood is only discovered by testing, it is called *microscopic hematuria*. Blood is not normally present in the urine. If blood is found, your doctor will try to determine the cause.

The most common cause of blood in the urine is an infection of the urinary tract. There are many other causes. Some of these other causes are particularly common in elderly patients. Anticoagulants (blood thinners) are an example of these other causes.

Important Points in Treatment

The treatment necessary, if blood is found in your urine, varies with the cause. Some causes of bleeding in the urine are serious, even life-threatening problems. Bleeding should be called to the attention of your doctor and evaluated.

Notify Our Office If

- You note blood in your urine.

Acetaminophen Interactions with the Kidney

Patient and Caregiver's Guide

General Information

Acetaminophen is a commonly used analgesic drug. It is used for headache and many other kinds of pain. Although it is usually identified with Tylenol, it is found in many other over-the-counter pain medications. Acetaminophen may have toxic effects on the liver and the kidneys. The dose of drug required to produce toxic effect is close to the dose used for treatment of pain. The usual tablet contains 500 mg of the drug. A dose of one tablet or capsule four times per day is not uncommon. A dose larger than two tablets or capsules four times per day comes close to the dose that can produce toxicity.

This medication is safe if used properly, with restrictions on the number of tablets or capsules taken daily. Patients who have abused alcohol may be unusually susceptible to the effects of this drug.

Important Points in Treatment

If you customarily use acetaminophen for the treatment of mild pain or headache, you should be careful to adhere to the recommended dosage guidelines. It is unwise to take more than 4 g of this drug in any day.

Notify Our Office If

- You believe that you have taken an excessive dose of acetaminophen. This is an urgent circumstance. If you cannot reach the office, go immediately to the emergency room.

Vaginitis

General Information

Inflammation involving the vagina is a common complaint in elderly women. The normal vaginal discharge decreases in quantity with aging, and it becomes less acidic. This discharge normally provides for self-cleansing, and the acidic nature of the discharge inhibits the possible growth of infecting organisms. After menopause, changes also occur in the vagina that increase susceptibility to infections. These changes result from a decrease in the amount of estrogen, the female hormone, that occurs after menopause.

The prime symptom of vaginitis is itching. It may be felt in or around the vagina. It is a persistent and bothersome symptom. Associated with the itching is a vaginal discharge that occasionally is bloody. If an infection occurs, the discharge may have an odor, and there may be swelling in the tissues surrounding the vagina.

Important Points in Treatment

Many topical medicines are available to treat any infection and to reverse the menopausal changes in the vagina. Your physician will select the medicine based on the probable type of infection and the degree of postmenopausal change.

It is best to wear all-cotton undergarments, which can help to keep the vaginal area dry. Sexual intercourse should be avoided while vaginitis is active.

Notify Our Office If

- You have itching or burning in the vagina.
- You have bloody vaginal discharge.

Sexuality

General Information

Sexual desire does not necessarily change with aging. Just as there are some younger people with low interest in sex and some with high, there are elders with variable interest. Desire may change with age *but not necessarily because of* the aging process. Some diseases of aging do interfere with potency or desire, but this is a secondary effect. Sexual desires, sexual capability, and sexual satisfaction remain important factors for many older people.

Matters of sexuality and sexual issues are highly personal, but they are also important issues of health and well-being. Your physician will help you find answers to questions concerning sexuality, and you need not refrain from discussing these issues. Your physician can arrange access to specialists and counseling for complex problems.

Men

If there is any aging component to sexuality, it is probably the slowing of arousal, and this occurs principally in men. This slowing does not impair sexual function. Although potency may decrease in men, there is no loss of fertility with aging. There is no physiological male climacteric or menopause.

Impotence (erectile dysfunction) can occur but not because of aging. Psychological factors are a primary factor in causing impotence, but usually it is not the sole factor. Alcohol and drug effects are also major causes. The most common diseases that can cause impotence are diabetes and vascular insufficiency. A host of other diseases are responsible for a few cases of impotence.

Women

Women have a clearly defined limit of fertility: menopause. However, there is no age limit to libido, and women generally continue their pattern of sexual activity into their elder years.

Menopausal changes in the vagina include dryness, which may increase susceptibility to infection and may cause some discomfort during intercourse. These are treatable problems. Illness imposes indirect limitations on a woman's sexual activity.

Male Impotence

Patient and Caregiver's Guide

General Information

Male impotence is the inability to maintain (or attain) a penile erection that is sufficient to permit sexual intercourse. It is distinguished from libido, which is sexual desire. The two function independently. Male impotence has many causes, and these increase in frequency with age. Difficulties with blood supply and neurologic changes are common causes of this dysfunction. Many drugs have impotence as a side effect, as does alcohol. The problem requires a thorough evaluation. The best treatment is treatment of the underlying problem where possible.

Important Points in Treatment

Treatment may involve medical therapy with drugs, surgical therapy on blood vessels, psychological treatment, or the use of drugs or mechanical devices to permit an erection. Your doctor will discuss the options that best address your problems and needs.

Psychological therapy, although effective, is useful in relatively few patients because psychologic problems are an uncommon cause of male impotence. Surgical therapy directed toward restoring blood flow has little use in the elderly patient.

Mechanical devices are of two categories. There are external devices that use a vacuum to cause tumescence, which is maintained by placing a restrictive ring around the base of the penis. Not all patients find this device effective and/or acceptable. When used, the restrictive ring should not be left in place for longer than a half hour. Implanted devices in the penis require surgery and are subject to complications, such as infection, pain, malfunction, and shortening of the penis. They are usually not offered unless nonsurgical techniques are ineffective.

Medical treatment may involve replacement of hormones when a hormone deficiency has caused the impotence or the use of drugs to promote tumescence. Some drugs (alprostadil, Caverject) may be delivered into the urethra or injected into the penis to cause the erection. These drugs have side effects and may cause scarring over time. Injections should not be used in patients on anticoagulants.

Several medications are approved for the treatment of impotence. These include sildenafil (Viagra), which acts directly on the muscles in blood vessels in the penis to promote erection when the individual is sexually stimulated, and vardenafil, which acts like sildenafil and tadalafil, which has a similar but longer effect. When an erection occurs, it lasts for 10 minutes. These drugs are not effective in all patients. The dose may need to be adjusted. There are few side effects. This class of drugs should not be used by patients taking nitrates for heart disease or alpha-blocking drugs such as those used to treat prostatic enlargement.

 ## Notify Our Office If

- You have experienced difficulty achieving or maintaining an erection.

Dyspareunia

General Information

Dyspareunia is painful intercourse. After menopause, there is a gradual atrophy of estrogen-dependent genital tissues. The tissues of the lower vagina, including the labia and the lower portion of the bladder and urethra, are involved.

The vagina undergoes some atrophy. It grows shorter and the lining thins. Secretions may decrease. These changes may result in pain during intercourse.

Important Points in Treatment

Supplemental estrogens can reverse some of these atrophic changes. In cases in which treatment with oral estrogen is unacceptable, topical preparations are available. Lubricants that are water soluble can also provide some comfort.

Notify Our Office If

- You experience painful intercourse.

CHAPTER 15

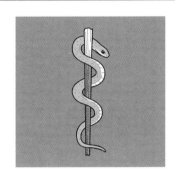
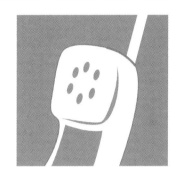

Temperature Regulation

Hypothermia

Patient and Caregiver's Guide ▪ ▪ ▪

General Information

Hypothermia is a decrease in body temperature to a level that is below normal. The normal metabolism and exercise of the human body produce heat. The body tries to save or lose this heat to keep the body's temperature within a narrow range.

The vascular system is the prime regulator of body temperature. Because of aging changes, it is possible for elderly patients to lose heat or to fail to conserve heat faster than at a younger age. Elderly patients are particularly susceptible to hypothermia.

Besides vascular changes, a number of other factors can contribute to hypothermia. Malnutrition, which can be thought of as lack of fuel, is one important factor. Changes in the central nervous system or the brain, such as those that occur in dementia, can impair one's ability to feel cold so that one does not take the protective actions necessary to warm up. Loss of the usual insulating layer of fat below the skin may be another factor.

Drugs, particularly sedatives and tranquilizers that can impair perception of cold, can lead to hypothermia. Any disease that decreases the ability to feel cold, impairs the response of the heart and the circulation, causes inactivity, or causes a decrease in exercise can also promote the development of hypothermia.

Normally, when a person chills, the response includes shivering, which is a kind of exercise of the muscles that promotes warming. Shivering is often absent in elderly patients with hypothermia. These patients feel cold not just in the extremities, which can be normal, but also in the trunk. They appear pale. As the cold progresses, it depresses bodily functions. Finally, coma may occur.

Important Points in Treatment

Prevention of hypothermia is always better than treatment. In the cold months, set the thermostat or heating control in your home to maintain the temperature at a minimum of 65°F. If you do not

---

353

have a thermostat, keep a reliable, readable thermometer where it can be easily checked regularly. Thermometers that have indicators or numbers that are difficult to read or that are kept in locations not likely to be visited offer little benefit in keeping track of the indoor temperature.

Hypothermia is a medical emergency. The patient needs to be rewarmed slowly and naturally. The patient is wrapped in blankets or a quilt, which permits the patient to rewarm himself or herself naturally.

Rapid rewarming of an elderly patient can cause profound changes in the heart and circulation and can result in death. If slow rewarming using only the natural mechanism fails, rapid rewarming using external heat needs to be done in a hospital intensive care setting.

Notify Our Office If

● You feel unusually cold.

Hyperthermia

General Information

Hyperthermia is an increase in body temperature to a level that is above normal. Fever as a result of infection is a form of hyperthermia. Abnormalities of the body's heat-regulating system can also produce hyperthermia at a time and in a setting that are inappropriate. Disorder of the heat-regulating system is a particular problem in elderly patients.

Normal body metabolism produces heat. The body loses this heat by radiation into the surrounding air and by the formation and evaporation of sweat to produce cooling. The heat loss is controlled by an increase or decrease of blood flow to the skin.

As the surrounding air gets warmer, such as in the summer, heat loss by radiation is less effective. When the humidity rises, evaporation of sweat becomes less effective as a mechanism for heat loss. These mechanisms may become even less effective as a result of age-related changes. In addition, the body's responses to heat, including the cooling mechanism, have to call on the heart and the vascular system to be effective. Heart disease, a common problem of elderly patients, may result in decreased effective heat regulation. Warm, humid summer days pose a high risk for hyperthermia for the susceptible elderly person.

- Heat cramps: Profuse sweating with loss of water and salt can result in *heat cramps*. These cramps may come on with sudden activity. Rest and replacement of water and salt prevent further cramps. With heat cramps, body temperature is normal.
- Heat exhaustion: Worsening water loss or salt loss can produce *heat exhaustion*. Patients become disoriented and have a loss of appetite. Nausea and vomiting may occur. As heat exhaustion worsens, the patient may become dizzy, light-headed, and faint. With heat exhaustion, body temperature is normal or elevated.
- Heat stroke: *Heat stroke*, a serious problem, occurs with high body temperatures. Fainting occurs often after dizziness or

other symptoms associated with heat exhaustion. Heart, brain, and kidney abnormalities may occur. Heat stroke is a medical emergency.

Important Points in Treatment

It is better to prevent problems of hyperthermia than to treat them. Appropriate dress and modification of exercise during warm weather are important steps. Cooling with fans or air conditioning can be an effective preventive measure.

Hyperthermia, particularly heat stroke, is a medical emergency. Cooling, which is essential, is carefully undertaken to prevent untoward changes in the vascular system. Treatment of heat cramps may require the use of salts and water administered by injection in the vein. Oral and sometimes intravenous fluids are used in the treatment of heat exhaustion.

Notify Our Office If

- You become light-headed or faint on warm, humid days.
- You have cramps, particularly on warm, humid days.

CHAPTER 16

 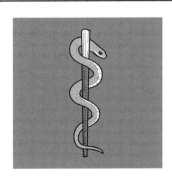 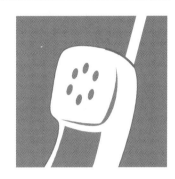

Rheumatic and Orthopedic Problems

Osteoporosis

Patient and Caregiver's Guide

General Information

Osteoporosis is one of several bone diseases that occurs with more frequency in elderly patients. It may occur in both men and women, but it is more common and begins somewhat earlier in women.

Osteoporosis is a decline in bone mass, that is, in the total amount of bone substance. As the bones lose calcium and become less dense, they are more susceptible to fracture. Trauma is not necessarily required to cause a fracture in an osteoporotic bone. Fractures may occur with no more stress than is created during the usual activities of daily living. These bones, of course, are easily fractured when trauma does occur.

There are several types of osteoporosis. The most common is post-menopausal osteoporosis, which physicians call *type I osteoporosis*. Less common is senile osteoporosis, called *type II osteoporosis* by physicians. In addition, many diseases and drugs can cause osteoporosis, called *secondary osteoporosis*. Types I and II osteoporosis are diseases of aging.

At greatest risk for osteoporosis are white or Asian women who have had early menopause or have undergone surgical removal of the ovaries. Other risk factors include a family history of the disease, an inactive lifestyle, poor nutritional intake of calcium, deficiency of vitamin D, and smoking. Some kinds of prescription drugs may predispose patients to develop osteoporosis. Osteoporosis usually remains a completely asymptomatic process until a bone breaks.

Diagnosis of osteoporosis is often made at the time of an x-ray examination performed for another purpose. Calcium content causes bones to show up on x-ray film. Osteoporotic bones are less dense. Bony changes, such as collapse of vertebrae or fractures, may also be apparent on x-ray examination.

Important Points in Treatment

Prevention of osteoporosis is far better than treatment of the established disease. A program of selected exercise, calcium supplements, and, in some women, hormone replacement can prevent osteoporosis. The same approach can afford some benefits to already involved bones. In some types of osteoporosis, vitamin D may be used as well. The diet should contain both adequate calcium and adequate calories. Supplemental calcium is often recommended. Selection of the proper patients for hormone or vitamin D therapy depends on the nature of the osteoporosis and the occurrence of other problems or risk factors. It is a decision that your physician will make with you. Patients with significant bone resorption may require anti-resorption therapy. The drugs for this have side effects, particularly related to irritation of the stomach and the lower portion of the esophagus (the swallowing tube). A number of other drugs are used in the treatment of osteoporosis.

It is possible to follow the effectiveness of the treatment with measurements of bone density. These measurements are usually carried out over a prolonged period because changes of the bone are slow to occur.

Fractures require specific management with splints, casts, bracing, and appropriate rehabilitation. The management selected depends on the nature of the fracture.

Notify Our Office If

- You have bone pain. Often the first indication of a broken bone in elderly patients is the sudden onset of bone pain.

Foot Problems

Patient and Caregiver's Guide

General Information

After a lifetime of walking on feet that are bound in ill-fitting shoes, several potential problems develop. Much can be done to avoid the difficulties that occur with the aging foot. Careful treatment and thoughtful selection of footwear can slow or arrest these changes. It is also possible to adapt to changes that are irreversible with proper footwear. This occasionally requires the use of prescription footwear.

Foot problems may also plague sufferers of several diseases that are common in elderly patients. Diabetes, arthritis, peripheral vascular disease, and heart disease, particularly with heart failure, may all cause foot problems.

When foot problems are complicated, a referral to a dermatologist, orthopedist, rheumatologist, neurologist, or podiatrist may be necessary.

Important Points in Treatment

Corns and calluses form where pressure from a shoe causes thickening of the skin. Careful selection and fitting of footwear that avoids pressure points should be made. Where established deformities cause pressure, foam or felt pads can redistribute the pressure and prevent the formation of corns and calluses. Your physician can pare thickened areas of skin. He or she can also prescribe footwear or appliances so that further trauma to these pressure points can be avoided.

Skin and nail problems may be due to dry skin or to fungus infection. Moisturizing creams that can soften and hydrate dry skin can help prevent further drying. If infections with skin fungus have occurred, medication may be needed. Chronic fungus infection, although unlikely to respond to simple athlete's foot therapy, can respond to some new prescription therapies. This is particularly true of infections that involve the toenails. The advice of a dermatologist or a podiatrist is sometimes needed.

Notify Our Office If

- You have the beginning of a horny or thickened area of skin over a bony prominence of your foot.
- The skin of your foot is persistently reddened or inflamed.

Fungus Infection of the Toenails

Patient and Caregiver's Guide ◼◼◼

General Information

Fungal infection involving the feet is a very common problem. This is usually called athlete's foot. Somewhat less frequently the fungal infection may occur in the toenail. This causes the toenail to thicken and become deformed. The deformity may press on the shoe and cause discomfort.

Infected toenails are a chronic problem that requires prolonged therapy. The therapeutic choice usually involves a year-long application of cream, a month-long treatment with an oral therapy, or surgical removal of the infected nail. All of these are effective forms of therapy, but they do require careful attention to keeping the feet clean and dry.

Important Points in Therapy

Toenails are very slow growing. Infections in these nails persist until the entire infected portion of the nail has grown out and is removed. This requires chronic therapy. Often this therapy is provided by a podiatrist. Before beginning therapy, cultures will be obtained from the nail to ensure that the problem is infection with a fungus.

Call Our Office If

- You notice that your nails have become thickened or deformed.

Osteoarthritis

Patient and Caregiver's Guide

General Information

Wear and tear on joints can produce the changes of osteoarthritis. The problem increases with each passing decade. Thus, osteoarthritis is a problem of elderly patients.

Joints move smoothly because there is a moist lining or membrane cushioned by underlying cartilage between the bones that form the joints. With the development of osteoarthritis, this cartilage cushion begins to deteriorate. Continued wear causes the underlying bone to change its shape, and this produces the arthritic deformity. Osteoarthritis is slowly progressive. The early changes of osteoarthritis may cause no symptoms. It does not involve all joints equally. The fingers and toes, knees, and spine and hips are particularly susceptible. With movement, joints are painful, but they recover and become pain free with rest. As the disease progresses, changes on x-ray studies become evident.

Pain is the most common symptom of osteoarthritis. The pain is worse with movement of the joint. It is usually relieved by rest. Joints may feel stiff in the morning. In some patients inflammation may occur in the damaged joint. The inflamed joint may be painful even at rest.

Important Points in Treatment

Anti-inflammatory drugs, when combined with physical therapy, can slow the progression of osteoarthritis and can help to restore function lost when joints are sore. Specific treatment may be useful for muscle spasm. Weight reduction is helpful in reducing the pain associated with the arthritis.

Sore, stiff joints pose major problems in carrying out the simple acts of daily living. It is difficult to tie shoes, unscrew lids, and work buttons and zippers. Many aids are available to help in the performance of daily chores. The best guidance to resources in your area is found in rehabilitation units. The professionals in these units have the skills to help you select among the many devices offered to obtain the items that are most appropriate for your particular needs.

Surgical treatment may be helpful for some patients. Replacement of joints requires major surgery. Discuss the risks and possible benefits with your physician.

Notify Our Office If

- You have sudden onset of joint soreness that cannot be explained by overuse or injury.
- You have a joint that is red, warm to the touch, swollen, or tender.

Arthritis of the Wrist and Hand

Patient and Caregiver's Guide

General Information

Wear and tear takes a toll on all of our joints; the joints used most are the most susceptible. Osteoarthritis is common in the wrist and hand. In addition to generalized arthritis, damage occurs in individual joints in the hand and wrist because of the frequent performance of a particular task. For example, knitting and crocheting are particularly hard on the joint at the base of the thumb.

Arthritic diseases other than osteoarthritis also commonly affect the hand and wrist. Rheumatoid arthritis occurs there. Gout may involve the hand and wrist as well.

Joint disease causes pain in the joint, with swelling, redness, and stiffness. Pain may be present only on motion or at rest as well. Report these signs and symptoms to your physician.

In addition, joint disease may cause inflammation of the tendons. Inflamed tendons also cause pain on motion and tenderness around the joint. Sometimes swelling and redness are also present. Occasionally, joints or tendons catch, and the joints may lack temporarily. Sometimes chronic changes become evident only after a minor injury.

Important Points in Treatment

The specific treatment for arthritis depends on its cause. Many general measures help control symptoms. Inflamed joints and tendons need rest. At the same time, joints particularly need to retain their full range of motion, and the muscles moving the joints need enough exercise to prevent muscle wasting and atrophy. Accomplish this by alternating periods of rest of the joint with careful exercise. Select exercises with your physician or a physical therapist.

Application of heat can be helpful in reducing pain and discomfort. Use heat carefully to avoid injuring tissues. This is not a case in which hotter is better. Patients with vascular disease must be particularly careful about the application of heat.

Anti-inflammatory drugs, administered either as pills or by injection, are used to improve the symptoms of pain and stiffness. Many powerful drugs are available without a prescription. These medications have serious side effects, some even with normal doses. The pharmacy may be an inexpensive source for these medicines, but your physician is still the best counsel regarding selection and dosage.

Notify Our Office If

- You have new onset of swelling or pain in a joint.
- You have locking of a joint when you try to move it.
- You have heat in a joint, particularly with fever or chills.
- You have dark stools or blood in your bowel movements, particularly if you are taking arthritis medicines.

Arthritis of the Knee

Patient and Caregiver's Guide ▪ ▪ ▪

General Information

Wear and tear take a toll on all of our joints; the joints used most are the most susceptible. Osteoarthritis is common in the knee. Other kinds of arthritis, such as rheumatoid arthritis and gout, can also affect the knee. The knee is subject to injury when a person participates in sports while young, but the effects are delayed for many years.

Proper function of the knee joint is important for walking, but it is also involved in rising from a chair and ascending stairs. Disability of the knee quickly comes to one's attention. The nature of the knee joint makes it susceptible to locking. This is often due to broken-off bits of bone or cartilage in the joint, called joint mice. Report sudden onset of pain or discomfort in the knee to your physician.

Important Points in Treatment

The specific treatment for arthritis depends on its cause. Many general measures help control symptoms. The knee is one of the major weight-bearing joints in the body. It benefits from rest, if inflamed. Rest for the knee includes freedom from weight bearing. If you are overweight, you will get an increment of benefit for each pound you lose. Weight loss is a slow process, but a weight-loss program should be started without delay.

The use of a cane or crutches can offer some immediate relief from weight bearing. There is always a safety factor to consider when using crutches. If not done carefully, the transfer of weight bearing from the leg to the arms and shoulders can cause the development of arthritic symptoms there as well. Instruction in the proper use of crutches is important to obtain the maximum benefit with the least risk of injury from falling. Adjust crutches to the right height and grip for their safe and effective use.

Use of a cane is simple, but it must be done properly to get the most relief from weight bearing. Instructions for cane use are available from a physical therapist, who can also help with the proper length of the cane, a feature important for maximum benefit in relief from weight bearing.

Joints need to retain their full range of motion, and the muscles moving the joints need enough exercise to prevent muscle wasting and atrophy. Accomplish this by alternating periods of rest of the joint with careful exercise. Select exercises with your physician or a physical therapist.

Application of heat can be helpful in reducing pain and discomfort. Use heat carefully to avoid injuring tissues. This is not a case in which hotter is better. Patients with vascular disease must be particularly careful about the application of heat.

Anti-inflammatory drugs, administered either as pills or by injection, are used to improve the symptoms of pain and stiffness. Many powerful drugs are available without a prescription. All of these medications have serious side effects, some even with normal doses. The pharmacy may be an inexpensive source for these medicines, but your physician is still the best counsel regarding selection and dosage.

Notify Our Office If

- You have new onset of pain in your knee.
- You have locking of the knee when you try to move it.
- You have heat in your knee, particularly with fever or chills.
- You have dark stools or blood in your bowel movements, particularly if you are taking arthritis medicines.

Knee Replacement

Patient and Caregiver's Guide

General Information

Arthritis of the knee can become an incapacitating health problem. Standing, walking, rising from a chair, and even sitting involve the knee. When the knee is painful, these activities are difficult; when the knee joint stiffens, some of these activities begin to be impossible. Surgical knee replacement should be considered when moving around and caring for yourself become too difficult.

Most knee replacements are done for knees affected by osteoarthritis. Replacement surgery is also performed on patients with other kinds of arthritis affecting the knee joint. Knee replacements may also be done in some cases of a broken knee.

The first consideration is your ability to undergo the surgery. Knee replacement is a major surgical procedure, but it is done on patients of all ages. Patients tolerate it well. Those who have other serious health problems may need additional evaluation to determine any additional risks they may incur.

Important Points in Treatment

- Knee replacement is a safe operation. Complications occur in less than 1% of patients.
- The replacement knee lasts between 10 and 15 years before it begins to show wear. Need for replacement is likely after about 10 years.
- Recovery from knee replacement surgery is a matter of gradual improvement in function over a period of months. Although the stay in the hospital may be short, an interval of physical rehabilitation is necessary before full recovery.
- Even with full recovery, some limitation of motion in the knee remains. Prosthetic joints cannot fully recapture all of the motion of a natural joint. A slight limp may persist.

Arthritis of the Hip

Patient and Caregiver's Guide

General Information

Wear and tear take a toll on all of our joints; the joints used most are the most susceptible. Osteoarthritis is common in the hip. Other kinds of arthritis, such as rheumatoid arthritis and gout, can also affect the hip. The hip is subject to injury. Hip fracture is a threat to elderly patients because of the thinning of the bone as a result of osteoporosis that occurs with aging. This thinning often involves the main supporting bone of the hip. Hence, fracture, with even minor trauma, tends to occur in the senior years.

Proper function of the hip joint is important for walking, but it is also involved in rising from a chair and ascending stairs. Disability of the hip quickly comes to one's attention. Report sudden onset of pain or discomfort in the hip to your physician.

Important Points in Treatment

The specific treatment for any arthritis depends on its cause. Many general measures help control symptoms. The hip is the major weight-bearing joint in the body. It benefits from rest, if inflamed. Rest for the hip includes freedom from weight bearing. If you are overweight, you will get an increment of benefit for each pound you lose. Weight loss is a slow process, but a weight-loss program should be started without delay.

The use of a cane or crutches can offer some immediate relief from weight bearing. There is always a safety factor to consider when using crutches. If not done carefully, the transfer of weight bearing from the hip to the arms and shoulders can cause the development of arthritic symptoms there as well. Instruction in the proper use of crutches is important to obtain the maximum benefit with the least risk of injury from falling. Adjust crutches to the right height and grip for their safe and effective use.

Use of a cane is simple, but it must be done properly to get the most relief from weight bearing. Instructions for cane use are available from a physical therapist, who can also help with the proper length of the cane, a feature important for maximum benefit in relief from weight bearing.

Joints need to retain their full range of motion, and the muscles moving the joints need enough exercise to prevent muscle wasting and atrophy. Accomplish this by alternating periods of rest of the joint with careful exercise. Select exercises with your physician or a physical therapist.

Application of heat can be helpful in reducing pain and discomfort. Use heat carefully to avoid injuring tissues. This is not a case in which hotter is better. Patients with vascular disease must be particularly careful about the application of heat.

Anti-inflammatory drugs, administered either as pills or by injection, are used to improve the symptoms of pain and stiffness. Many powerful drugs are available without a prescription. All of these medications have serious side effects, some even with normal doses. The pharmacy may be an inexpensive source for these medicines, but your physician is still the best counsel regarding selection and dosage.

Notify Our Office If

- You have new onset of pain in your hip.
- You have locking of the hip when you try to move it.
- You have heat in your hip, particularly with fever or chills.
- You have dark stools or blood in your bowel movements, particularly if you are taking arthritis medicines.

Hip Replacement

Patient and Caregiver's Guide

General Information

Arthritis of the hip can become an incapacitating health problem. Standing, walking, rising from a chair, and even sitting involve the hip. When the hip is painful, these activities are difficult; when the hip joint stiffens, some of these activities begin to be impossible. Surgical hip replacement should be considered when moving around and caring for yourself become too difficult.

Most hip replacements are done for hips affected by osteoarthritis. Replacement surgery is also performed on patients with other kinds of arthritis affecting the hip joint. Hip replacements may also be done in some cases of a broken hip.

The first consideration is your ability to undergo the surgery. Hip replacement is a major surgical procedure, but it is done on patients of all ages. Patients tolerate it well. Those who have other serious health problems may need additional evaluation to determine any additional risks they may incur.

Important Points in Treatment

- Hip replacement is a safe operation. Complications occur in less than 1% of patients.
- The replacement hip lasts between 10 and 15 years before it begins to show wear. Need for replacement is likely after about 10 years.
- Recovery from hip replacement surgery is a matter of gradual improvement in function over a period of months. Although the stay in the hospital may be short, an interval of physical rehabilitation is necessary before full recovery.
- Even with full recovery, some limitation of motion in the hip remains. Prosthetic joints cannot fully recapture all of the motion of a natural joint. A slight limp may persist.

Gout

General Information

Gout is a cause of acute joint pain and occurs at an earlier age in men than in women. Patients with gout have elevations in the blood of a component called *uric acid*. Most often these elevations occur because the kidney fails to excrete the uric acid as fast as it is made. Gradually, crystals of uric acid deposit in the tissues. These deposits occur around joints, and the release of the crystals into the joint may cause the sudden development of arthritis. The joint becomes red, swollen, hot, and tender. The tenderness is extreme, and patients with fully developed gouty attacks are unable to sustain even a light touch on the joint, such as from clothing or bedclothes.

Without treatment, the arthritis lasts several days to a week. Usually, gout affects one joint at a time, although attacks involving several joints do occur. Classically, gout is associated with the joint in the great toe, but any joint may be involved.

If attacks recur, chronic arthritis may develop in the involved joint. Often deposits of uric acid, called *tophi,* distort and interfere with the smooth function of the joint. Tophi may also occur in other tissues, such as in the ear. Uric acid deposition can also cause kidney stones.

Your physician can often suspect the diagnosis of gout based on your history and the appearance of the inflamed joint. Blood tests may show an elevation in uric acid. If there is uncertainty about the diagnosis, fluid from the joint is tested for the presence of uric acid crystals.

Important Points in Treatment

The treatment of acute attacks of gouty arthritis is with anti-inflammatory drugs or a drug called *colchicine*. Once the acute arthritis is controlled, long-term treatment to block the production of uric acid may prevent further attacks and will protect the kidneys from the development of kidney stones as well.

Notify Our Office If

- You have sudden onset of a painful, red, or swollen joint.

Polymyalgia Rheumatica

Patient and Caregiver's Guide

General Information

The combination of pain and stiffness in the shoulders and upper arms and in the hips and thighs occurs in a disease called *polymyalgia rheumatica*. This disease usually affects people over age 50. This pain is persistent and progressive and can cause substantial disability. Weight loss and fever may also occur. There may be limitation of motion of involved muscles and joints. Involved shoulder and thigh muscles may be tender. Up to one fourth of patients with polymyalgia rheumatica also have a problem called *temporal arteritis*. This presents with symptoms of headache and has the potential for causing more severe complications, such as blindness.

Important Points in Treatment

The use of medications called *corticosteroids* produces remarkable and rapid improvement in this disease. The required dose may be large enough to produce side effects. Careful follow-up with your physician is mandatory to ensure that you are receiving the maximum benefit from the drug with the minimum possibility of damage. Once the symptoms are controlled, therapy at a lower dose may be continued for a long period to suppress the disease and prevent its return.

Giant Cell Arteritis (Temporal Arteritis)

Patient and Caregiver's Guide

General Information

When inflammation occurs in the large blood vessels, the arteries that run beneath the skin on the temporal (temple) areas of the head, the disease is temporal arteritis. Frequency of occurrence increases with aging. It often occurs in association with a problem called *polymyalgia rheumatica*. Temporal arteritis presents with throbbing headaches. These headaches occur in the area of the involved artery. Most often this is along the temples, but the arteries in the front and back of the neck and in the eye may be involved as well. The pain tends to be throbbing and occurs in rhythm with the pulse. When the arteries in the eye become involved, partial blindness may occur. There is an increased risk of the development of an aneurysm (dilation) of the aorta in the abdomen. An annual examination may be suggested to watch for this possible complication.

Important Points in Treatment

Treatment with corticosteroids is highly effective in controlling the disease, including the prevention of blindness. The doses used are large, and some side effects are possible. Risks must be balanced against benefits. Treatment with steroids may continue for up to a year.

Notify Our Office If

- You experience a change in vision associated with headache.
- You experience throbbing headaches, particularly involving the side of the head.
- You experience onset of tenderness in the temples.

Muscle Cramps

Patient and Caregiver's Guide

General Information

Although of unknown cause, muscle cramps are a frequent problem in elderly patients. Cramps can occur because of electrolyte abnormalities, but more commonly an idiopathic or unexplained variety of leg cramp is the problem in older patients. These muscle spasms occur at night and awaken an individual from a sound sleep. Muscle cramps, commonly called *charley horses,* may occur at any age. They often follow exercise or prolonged posture in an unusual position. Although these cramps may have a similar effect, they differ in cause from the cramps that occur in the elderly.

Important Points in Treatment

One can relieve a leg cramp by standing and placing the involved muscle under some tension. The need to do this disturbs the night's sleep.

Cramps can be prevented with a nightly dose of medication. It is most common to use quinine, although other medications may be effective. Chronic use of these medications can lead to side effects, and they should be used under the direction of your physician. Physical therapy may help, particularly if you do the prescribed exercises just before bedtime.

The best management for cramps that result from metabolic abnormalities and renal disease is treatment of the underlying problem.

Notify Our Office If

- You get night cramps in the leg or foot.
- You have frequent muscle cramps unrelated to exercise or tension.

CHAPTER 17

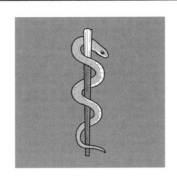
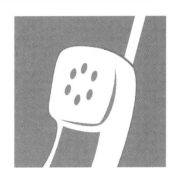

Skin Problems

Pressure Sores

Patient and Caregiver's Guide

General Information

Pressure sores, also called *bedsores* and *decubitus ulcers,* occur when there is unrelenting pressure on the skin. This pressure interferes with blood flow, thus causing the skin to break down and form an ulcer. Any diseases or problems that lead to immobility can result in pressure sores. It is a common secondary problem in elderly patients.

Pressure points naturally occur over bony prominences or in areas where the bone is just beneath the skin, uncushioned by surrounding muscles and fat. Skin is also more susceptible to breakdown, if it becomes wet and macerated. Friction caused by clothes against skin, skin against skin, or tugging and pulling on skin is a shearing force, which may also cause the skin to break down.

The first indication of a bedsore is an area that is red but that pales (blanches) on touch. Common sites are over the pelvic area, the back, the outside of the hips, the heels, the bones on each side of the ankle, the elbows, and the back of the head. At the reddening stage, these changes are reversible.

All subsequent changes involve skin breakdown and the development of ulceration. If not attended to, the problem becomes one of successively deeper penetration of the ulcer. Secondary infections are common, spreading the damage and slowing the healing process.

Important Points in Treatment

Prevention of bedsores is the primary focus of attention. Passive movements are necessary for patients who cannot move themselves. It is best to set a 2-hour limit on resting without a position change. Even small bodily movements can help. A patient with only limited mobility may still make small adjustments in position that permit redistribution of the pressure placed on the skin, and this goes a long way toward the prevention of bedsores. Bony prominences need particular protection. Egg crate–like foam mattresses are a help in adjusting the distribution of pressure. Cushions made of similar material should be used when the patient is sitting for prolonged periods. These should replace pillows, which lack the ability to shift the focus of pressure. Rubber rings are not safe; they cut off circulation to the area inside the ring and can worsen bedsores. Sheepskin protectors (with the fleece on) for heels and elbows can be effective.

A variety of mattresses and beds designed to prevent bedsores are available. These can be expensive. Discuss any planned purchase with the patient's physician to be sure that the mattress selected is appropriate for the patient's problem and setting.

Good nutrition and scrupulous personal hygiene can help in keeping the skin clean and dry. This reduces the risk of ulceration. Patients with incontinence should have this problem addressed directly because the maceration caused may advance the problem of bedsores.

If ulcers occur, their management requires careful nursing care. A formal management program that fits the patient's setting and problem should be set up with the help of the patient's physician and the participation of health care services.

Notify Our Office If

- The patient has any skin breakdown, particularly in areas over bony prominences.

Contact Dermatitis

Patient and Caregiver's Guide

General Information

The skin may become inflamed because of contact with a variety of materials. Materials to which the patient is allergic or that are particularly irritating can induce an inflammatory response in the skin. Skin gradually acquires allergic sensitivity, and this becomes more common with aging. Aging changes in the skin also include thinning, which results in a more fragile and a less protected skin. These changes increase the susceptibility to irritants in elderly patients.

Irritant dermatitis is more common than allergic dermatitis. Both the home and the workplace are host to an increasing number of chemical agents with irritant potential. New agents should be introduced into the home or workplace cautiously to allow the identification of possible irritants that can cause dermatitis. When the use of irritant compounds is necessary, some protection can be afforded by wearing rubber gloves.

Allergic contact dermatitis is highly specific for each individual and each compound. Almost everything we contact can cause a skin rash. The only practical management is avoidance.

Important Points in Treatment

When a contact dermatitis skin rash occurs, keep the area clean and dry and allow the dermatitis to resolve on its own. Occasionally, a steroid cream is needed to reduce the skin inflammation and promote healing.

For recurrent or persistent dermatitis, your physician may refer you to a dermatologist for special testing to attempt to identify the offending compound.

Notify Our Office If

- You have sudden onset of a skin rash that fails to subside within a week.

Dry Skin

General Information

Aging of the skin produces changes in the glands that open through the pores onto the skin surface. Atrophy of these glands reduces the moisture that the skin retains in the dead and dying cells that form the outer layer of the skin.

With a seasonal drop in humidity, such as the one that occurs in winter, dry skin worsens. The dry air of central heating systems adds to the problem of dry skin. Exposure outdoors to the wind and cold is an additional factor.

Dry skin is easy to recognize by its scaly appearance and flaking. Often cracking occurs, and these cracks may become inflamed or secondarily infected. These cracks are portals for the entrance of irritants, such as cosmetics, soaps, and lint from clothing, causing further inflammation.

Important Points in Treatment

Humidify the air in your home as much as possible, particularly during the drier months. If use of a central humidifier is not possible, portable humidifiers can humidify one or two rooms. One should humidify the bedroom first, followed by the most used room in the home. The traditional trick of placing an open jar or can of water on the radiator or by a heating vent can help add to the humidity in the room.

Avoid drying agents. These include harsh soaps, alcohol-based scents, and alcohol-based lotions. Wash no more often than is necessary. After bathing, apply moisturizing lotions while the skin is still damp. It is helpful to use moisturizers after hand washing or before going outside into the dry cold.

Notify Our Office If

- You have sudden onset of a skin rash that fails to subside within a week.

Itching

General Information

An itch is a skin sensation. The other skin sensations are touch, pain, heat, and cold. An itch leads to a desire to scratch. Itching has many causes, from simple dryness of the skin to serious systemic diseases.

When itching is persistent or recurrent, the scratching that it leads to may cause injury to the skin. Often the injury itself produces further itching and a vicious cycle occurs.

Your physician will attempt to identify the cause or causes of the itching. If a cause can be identified, treatment of the cause, if possible, is the best way to control the itching. If the cause is not identifiable, your doctor may be able to prescribe medicines to help reduce the itch. It may also be necessary to treat the injury caused by scratching.

Important Points in Treatment

Do not scratch. If you cannot control the urge then use your finger tip, not the nail, to rub gently on the itching area. Use a good moisturizing lotion, particularly after a bath or shower. If itching persists, seek help from your physician.

Call Our Office If

- You develop a persistent or recurrent itch.
- Scratching produces a rash or other inflammation of the skin.

Sun-Exposed Skin

Patient and Caregiver's Guide ▪ ▪ ▪

General Information

The skin and its appendages, principally the hair and the nails, are susceptible to aging. The most common of all of the aging changes, gray hair, is an example of a skin appendage change. Many factors may affect the speed of the aging process in the skin. Exposure to sunlight speeds aging changes in the skin more than any other factor.

Aging of the skin produces thinning with some loss of pigmentation. The skin decreases in flexibility, and it may become more fragile and bruise more easily. The blood vessels in the skin may become dilated and visible. These are called *telangiectases*. Some hair loss may occur, and sweating may decrease. The skin becomes drier. Wrinkling becomes prominent.

Some of these changes seem to be accelerated with sun exposure. Sun exposure may produce spots of intense *pigmentation,* often called "liver spots," and areas of thickening called *keratoses*. Sunlight exposure is called *actinic* exposure. It may induce the development of cancer.

Important Points in Treatment

Preventive measures should begin in childhood with limitation of sun exposure. Protection with clothing, hats, sunscreens, and behavioral modification should become the norm. Most of us grew up at a time when a "healthy" tan was desired and sought. As a result, substantive damage from sun exposure has already occurred for most elderly patients. This is only minimally reversible, but further damage can be prevented by adopting protection against sun exposure. It is never too late to begin a program of sun protection to limit further damage.

Improvement in skin changes can occur with skin protection. Some kinds of changes from sun exposure improve with the use of tretinoin. The degree of improvement is limited, but it is real. This preparation has side effects. You should consult your physician for its use.

Herpes Zoster (Shingles)

Patient and Caregiver's Guide

General Information

Shingles is an infection caused by the same virus that produces chickenpox. After childhood, the chickenpox virus remains in nerves in a dormant state. If immunity to the virus wanes, the infection may become reactivated, producing a painful skin eruption commonly called *shingles*. This relapse has its peak occurrence between the ages of 50 and 70 years.

Although there may be many systemic symptoms, such as fever, chills, and malaise, pain is the most common feature. The skin rash, which starts as a raised, reddened area, may not appear for days after the onset of the pain. The rash quickly evolves into blister-like vesicles, permitting a diagnosis and explanation for the pain.

An attack of herpes zoster may be followed by prolonged pain in the affected area. Involvement of the eye may occur in some patients. There is a risk of blindness.

Important Points in Treatment

If consultation with your physician is early enough, treatment with an antiviral drug can shorten the course of the infection. This therapy is less effective if started 3 or more days after the onset of symptoms. Clean, wet compresses help keep the rash clean and free of secondary infection.

Secondary infection may require treatment with antibiotics. Except when the area of the rash is being treated with a compress, it should be kept clean and dry. The skin lesions contain the virus and can transmit chickenpox to people not previously exposed. Aspirin or acetaminophen (Tylenol) relieves much of the discomfort associated with the rash. Your physician should be consulted if severe pain persists.

Complications

The nerves of the face and of the eye can be involved. Report pain in the eye or the presence of lesions on the face, particularly the nose, to your physician immediately. Infection in these areas may require referral to an ophthalmologist or to an otolaryngologist for specialized care.

In most patients, the infection remains confined to the distribution of one or two nerves. In a few patients, particularly those with a disturbed immune system, the infection can spread and become diffuse. In selected patients who are highly susceptible, such as those receiving some kinds of cancer treatment or transplant recipients, treatment should begin at the onset to prevent the spread of the infection. Your physician will counsel you if this becomes necessary.

A few patients experience continued pain after the infection has healed. Report continued pain to your physician to allow proper therapy for its control.

Notify Our Office If

- You have blisters on your face or eye pain.
- Your blisters seem to spread.
- Pain persists after the rash has healed.
- The rash suddenly seems to become inflamed or infected and you have symptoms such as fever.

Fungal Infections
Patient and Caregiver's Guide ■ ■ ■

General Information

As the skin ages, it loses some of the defensive mechanisms involved in preventing fungal infection. Fungi that infect the skin are not particularly virulent, and they need breakdowns in the normal skin defenses to invade successfully.

Dry, healthy skin is resistant to fungal infection. Moist skin, particularly in a warm environment, creates a hothouse effect, within which fungi can flourish.

Important Points in Treatment
Feet

The feet are particularly susceptible to fungal infection at any age. This infection is called *tinea pedis,* or athlete's foot. Warm, sweaty feet in shoes rarely cleaned on the inside provide an optimum growth environment for fungi.

Prevention is best. Good foot care includes wearing clean socks, cleaning and drying the feet carefully, and using foot powder. If infections occur, the same basic foot care is essential. In addition, antifungal agents, such as creams, powders, or lotions, can clear up the infection. If the toenail becomes infected, oral medications for prolonged periods may be necessary.

Nails

Fungi that infect the skin may also infect the nails. This is called *tinea unguium.* The infection causes the nail to thicken and become distorted. Toenails can be painful, and a larger shoe may have to be worn.

Toenails are more often involved than fingernails. Nails grow slowly, and toenails notoriously so. Treatment of nail infection involves taking antifungal medication for long enough to allow all of the infected nail to grow out. This may take 18 months to 2 years for the toenails. Even with prolonged therapy, recurrence is common. Management of thickened and distorted nails by a podiatrist may be effective in relieving discomfort. Surgical removal of the nail may be an option.

Fungal Infection of the Groin

The other common site for fungal infection is the groin. This is called *tinea cruris*. The groin area is often a high-humidity region that promotes fungal growth. Keeping this area clean and dry with powder and careful selection of clothing is the best prevention and, if infection occurs, is an effective therapy.

Besides keeping the groin area clean and dry, a variety of effective topical creams are available. Your physician can help you select the most appropriate agent.

Complications

Patients with diseases, such as diabetes, are at risk for fungal infections. Patients who have some interference with immune responses, including patients with acquired immunodeficiency syndrome (AIDS), transplant recipients, patients receiving cancer chemotherapy, and patients receiving steroids, need to be unusually scrupulous about their personal hygiene to reduce the possibility of fungal infection. Avoid sharing nail-cutting instruments to prevent the passing of infection.

Notify Our Office If

- You develop itching of the feet and/or toes.
- You develop irregular marks on fingernails or toenails.
- You develop an itch in the groin area.

Hair Loss (Baldness)

Patient and Caregiver's Guide

General Information

Gradual loss of hair with aging is a common phenomenon. It is usually more apparent in men with shorter haircuts but can occur in women as well. The loss may involve the vertex (the top of the head) or the frontal areas just above the forehead on either side of the head. Baldness with aging should be distinguished from male pattern baldness. This is the gradual loss of hair from the forehead back to the vertex, which is the common form of baldness in younger men. Male pattern baldness is inherited.

Other sorts of baldness or hair loss may range from the loss of simple spots of hair *(alopecia areata)* to total hairlessness *(alopecia totalis)*. Baldness of this sort is not a function of aging, although it may occur in the elderly as well as in the young. There is also hair loss associated with the administration of drugs. Chemotherapy for the treatment of cancer is the most common cause. This sort of hairlessness is temporary. Hair growth usually returns after the cessation of the drug treatment.

Hair loss may also be associated directly with some diseases rather than their treatment. Your physician will evaluate you for possible causes of the hair loss.

Important Points in Treatment

The gradual hair loss that occurs with aging is thus far not preventable. This hair loss is accelerated by damage to the hair. Harsh treatment of your hair ranging from tight braids or hairdos through chemical treatments to bleach, dye, and curling can accelerate natural hair loss.

There are three options for hair loss. One is to ignore it. This is by far the most common and safest option. The second option is to disguise the hair loss. There are a wide variety of choices; however, most involve hair pieces. Little can be said about this option except that one should be a prudent purchaser. Deal with professionals of established reputation. Understand thoroughly what you are purchasing before you contract for the purchase.

The third option involves medical approaches to restoration or regrowth of hair. You should be aware that there are many non-medical (cosmetic) claims for shampoos, tonics, and other aids that will restore (rejuvenate) hair growth. These generally lack scientific medical evaluation or credibility, and a prospective buyer/user must evaluate the claims carefully before purchase. Current medical approaches to hair restoration or regrowth involve either hair transplantation or drugs to stimulate hair growth.

Hair transplantation is a surgical procedure in which skin containing hair follicles is moved from one part of the body to another. In its new location, the transplanted hair continues to flourish. A potential user needs to know that this is a cosmetic procedure and is usually not covered by health insurance. Evaluate the costs carefully. The individual transplants are small, and it takes many transplants to restore significant hair to a bald spot. Evaluate thoroughly the number of sessions that may be necessary.

The drugs currently offered for promotion of hair growth are minoxidil (Rogaine) and finasteride (Propecia). Propecia is useful only in men. It has an effect in young men but has not been useful for the elderly. Rogaine is available for both men and women; however, the stronger doses are for men only. The side effects of Rogaine are cardiovascular; thus, its use in elderly patients may be limited.

Notify Our Office If

- You notice unusual hair loss.
- You wish to consider drug treatment to restore hair growth.

CHAPTER 18

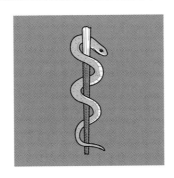
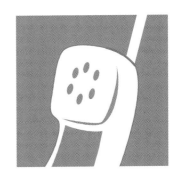

Surgery in the Elderly

Surgery in the Elderly

Patient and Caregiver's Guide

General Information

Many aging processes may increase the risk of surgery. Whether this increased risk is acceptable depends on the nature of the problem prompting the surgery. If it is an acute, life-threatening circumstance for which there are few or no alternatives, a high degree of risk may be acceptable in solving the problem. If the problem is not urgent and involves an elective procedure, it may be more appropriate to delay surgery until control of complicating factors reduces the risks as low as possible.

There is no specific age for the development of unusual risks at the time of surgery. In addition to a chronologic age, everyone also has a physiologic age, that is, the degree to which the various aging processes have actually progressed. For example, if the aging process in one person has reached a particular point at his or her chronologic age of 65, and another person does not reach that same point of age-related changes until age 75, then, although there is a difference of 10 years in their chronologic age, both have the same physiologic age. Problems and complications related to surgery vary with the physiologic age.

Most elderly patients, unless they have severe medical problems, can tolerate even major surgical procedures. The risk does increase, even in people of younger physiologic age, when two or more procedures must be done within a short time. If possible, it is better that there be a long interval between surgical procedures to keep the risks of the surgeries as low as possible.

Surgical risks always seem to be higher for individuals who must undergo an emergency procedure than for those who choose the time of their procedure. However, the increased risk for an emergency procedure is probably related to the medical problems and complications causing the emergency rather than to the procedure itself. Without complicating diseases or other problems, emergency surgery may not be any greater risk than elective surgery.

Your physician can help you select from the various surgical options. For many problems, surgical procedures have now been developed that are simpler to perform and less traumatic for the patient.

Inguinal Hernia

Patient and Caregiver's Guide

General Information

Inguinal hernias, or hernias that occur in the groin, may become evident at any age. Elderly patients are not particularly susceptible to, or particularly protected from, this problem. An inguinal hernia is the protrusion of a loop or more of the intestine through a weakened area in the abdominal wall. Increased intra-abdominal pressure, usually a result of straining, causes this protrusion.

Unless it is very large, a hernia represents only a potential problem instead of an immediate difficulty. The potential problem is that of a loop of intestine becoming entrapped in the hernia, called *incarceration*. On occasion, this trapped loop of intestine may become squeezed and the blood supply cut off, with the possibility of perforation of the intestinal wall. This is called *strangulation*. Strangulation usually results in obstruction of flow down the intestine. Should a perforation occur, it causes infection in the abdominal cavity, called *peritonitis*. Complications of this sort are true surgical emergencies that threaten the life of the individual. Controversy regarding the treatment of hernias has to do with when and how to repair the defect in the abdominal wall, if there are no complications. All hernias should be repaired, if the patient's other medical problems do not present an unusual risk.

Important Points in Treatment

Hernia repair is by operation with the use of a general anesthetic or with simple local anesthetic applied only to desensitize the area of the surgery. If the hernia is without complications and not large, it is possible for this sort of operation to be done as 1-day surgery on an outpatient basis. Short-stay surgery provides for rapid rehabilitation of the patient and decreases the possibility of other complications that occur after surgery, such as the development of blood clots in the legs. The ability of a patient to tolerate 1-day surgery is, in part, related to the presence of other health problems. Your physician is your best guide.

Notify Our Office If

- You have a hernia that is always present.
- You have pain or tenderness in a hernia.

Laparoscopic Surgery

Patient and Caregiver's Guide

General Information

Many kinds of surgery can now be performed using an instrument called a *laparoscope*. This instrument is inserted into the abdominal cavity through a small, half-inch, incision. The procedure may be done with minimal anesthetic. Other instruments may also be inserted through small incisions to perform the operation.

Operations that are commonly performed through the laparoscope include removal of the gallbladder, removal of the appendix, removal of a kidney, repair of a hernia, and treatment of reflux disease involving the esophagus (the swallowing tube). The laparoscope may also be used to look into the abdominal cavity when the diagnosis is uncertain. It is possible to biopsy (sample) the liver or other tissues through the laparoscope.

Although laparoscopic surgery is much less invasive than conventional surgery, it is not proper for all operations. In some cases where surgery can usually be done through the laparoscope, the surgeon may decide on the basis of what is seen that the operation needs to be converted to a conventional open surgery procedure. Often this occurs, if there has been previous surgery that has left adhesions or scars that prevent proper vision through the laparoscope.

The recovery after laparoscopic surgery is often rapid, and patients may leave the hospital on the day of surgery or on the next day. There is still a period of recuperation at home. Because this kind of surgery is less invasive, it is often suggested for the elderly.

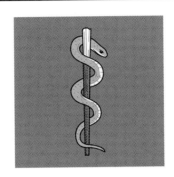
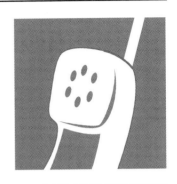

Infections

HIV and AIDS

Patient and Caregiver's Guide ▪ ▪ ▪

General Information

Acquired immunodeficiency syndrome (AIDS) and its antecedent infection human immunodeficiency virus (HIV) do occur in elderly patients. Most often HIV infection in this population is a result of having received a blood transfusion or blood products that contained the virus before proper screening measures were developed. It is important to remember that discovery of HIV infection does not imply that there is an immediate or inevitable threat of the development of AIDS. HIV is a chronic infection that develops slowly in many patients, taking years or a decade or more to progress.

The AIDS patients most often brought to our attention by the news media are those who have progressed to the advanced stages of the disease. Sensitive diagnostic tests for HIV infection now reveal that HIV-infected individuals often have long intervals with few or no symptoms. Although eventual progression to AIDS is common, it is not inevitable.

The question most often asked by the asymptomatic patient in whom HIV infection is diagnosed is how long it will take for AIDS to develop. There is no reliable answer. Excellent studies exist on the average interval of development, but this average cannot be accurately converted to a prediction for an individual patient. The patient's physician will obtain periodic laboratory tests that may help identify progression of the disease before symptoms and complications occur.

Important Points in Treatment

During the asymptomatic interval, the patient should continue his or her normal activities. The only restrictions are for activities that might lead to possible transmission of the virus to others. HIV is not spread by casual contact. The spread is by exposure to infected blood or other bodily fluids. Common usage of eating utensils, china, glassware, and bedding does not cause transmission of the virus. Quarantine is not necessary.

A few activities of daily living are a potential risk. HIV-infected individuals should not share razors, toothbrushes, or manicure tools, for instance, because these may contact blood and may cause injury to skin or mucous membranes. Common sense is a good guide. If an implement causes skin abrasions or bleeding, it should not be shared. Direct, unprotected sexual contact is also high-risk behavior.

A search continues for drugs for the early, asymptomatic stages of HIV infection to arrest or delay progression to AIDS. All drugs, whether experimental or approved, should be used under the direction of a physician in a proper and ethical manner.

Candidiasis (Yeast Infection)

Patient and Caregiver's Guide

General Information

Yeasts are not often a cause of infection. These organisms are not highly invasive. However, in patients who have some interference with defense mechanisms, yeast can gain a foothold and can cause disease. Aging changes in the skin, the vagina, and the oropharynx (the mouth and throat) offer opportunities for yeast to become infective. Diseases such as diabetes, HIV infection, and cancer may increase susceptibility to yeast infection. Treatment that interferes with immunity, such as steroid therapy or cancer chemotherapy, also increases susceptibility to this infection.

Yeast thrives in a warm, moist environment. Any location where skin surfaces come together for prolonged intervals are at risk. The axillae (armpits), the groin area, under the breasts, and within folds of fat are potential sites for infection with yeast.

The vagina, as it ages, loses some resistance to infection and becomes a more susceptible site for yeast infection. Although the mouth and throat are warm, moist areas, they are usually free of yeast because of the protective interaction with bacteria that compete with and suppress yeast growth. When the patient receives an antibiotic that interferes with the normal bacteria in the mouth and throat, yeast infection may become apparent. The infection may extend into the esophagus (the swallowing tube).

Important Points in Treatment

Yeast infection on the skin or in the vagina is treated with topical agents applied as a lotion or as a douche or suppository, respectively. Infection in the mouth or esophagus is treated with anti-yeast drugs in a mouthwash or a troche. Dentures and mouth appliances should be cleaned carefully to prevent them from reinfecting the mouth. Systemic drugs given by mouth or injection may be used to treat severe yeast infection.

Influenza

Patient and Caregiver's Guide

General Information

Influenza (flu) is a viral infection that occurs worldwide. It is primarily an infection of the lungs, nose, and throat. Each year the virus that causes this infection changes slightly, and it may change enough to allow even those people who have had a previous infection and who are immune to the earlier virus to become infected again. Infections may occur any time of the year, but they are most common in the fall and winter.

Although influenza infection does not respect any age group, the effects of the infection are more severe in elderly patients. The gradual process of aging affects the lungs and makes it easier for simple flu infections to become complicated by the development of pneumonia.

It is better to prevent influenza than to treat it. Excellent vaccines are available for the prevention of this infection. Because the virus changes yearly, annual revaccination with the current strain of influenza virus is important to keep up one's level of protection.

Important Points in Treatment

Older patients with influenza should see a physician. It is often difficult at the beginning of illness to tell a common cold from influenza infection. They share many common upper respiratory tract symptoms, such as runny nose, congestion, and sore throat. Infections that cause fever, chills, muscle aches and pains, and cough are suspected of being influenza. If these signs and symptoms develop, or if symptoms persist for more than 3 days, it is wise to consult your physician. If influenza is diagnosed early enough, it is possible to treat it with an antiviral drug that can shorten the period of illness. Two drugs are currently approved for the treatment of influenza, but they must be started within 48 hours of the beginning of the illness. These drugs may also be used as a preventive at the time of immunization to protect the patient while the immunization has time to take effect. In addition, there are inhaled drugs available for this same purpose.

Patients with uncomplicated influenza are most often treated at home. Bedrest is important to preserve one's full strength to oppose the infection. Your physician can recommend the best medication to lower the fever. (Remember, many medications interact in dangerous ways.) It is important to drink extra amounts of fluid. Fever can cause extra loss of fluid, and enough is needed to keep your kidneys working and healthy. Your physician will advise you about the best preparation for treatment of the cough.

As the infection and its symptoms subside, there should be a gradual return to usual activities. Full recovery may take several weeks. Early resumption of full activity may cause a relapse.

Notify Our Office If

- You have a sudden rise in temperature.
- You have a sudden worsening in breathing, with rapid breaths.
- You stop urinating.
- You have confusion or difficulty walking.

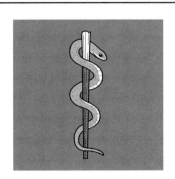
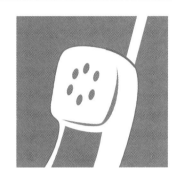

Paget's Disease of Bone

Paget's Disease of Bone

Patient and Caregiver's Guide

General Information

Paget's disease *(osteitis deformans)* occurs with increasing frequency with each decade of age. It is not equally common worldwide, seeming instead to have a predilection for the populations of English-speaking countries. It is a disease of unknown cause.

Paget's disease affects bone and may be limited to one bone or involve many. The most common sites affected are skull, clavicle (collar bone), and long bones of the arm and leg. The disease process causes reabsorption of bone, a change that is visible on x-ray examination. The disease may occur without causing any symptoms, and it is common to discover the problem when the patient undergoes x-ray examination for another purpose.

When the bony changes do cause symptoms, they can include headache, changes in hearing and balance, and visible deformities of the involved bones. The enlarging bones can occasionally cause pressure on nerves, which, in turn, can cause pain and other neurologic symptoms. If bones in the legs become involved, bowing of these bones can occur. Occasionally, the bones become fragile enough that a fracture occurs.

The changes in the bone increase the flow of blood through the bone. Occasionally, this can be so marked that it can be felt as warmer skin overlying the affected bone. This increase in blood flow can also produce strain on the heart and, in exceptional circumstances, can produce heart failure.

Important Points in Treatment

Patients who have no symptoms usually do not require treatment. Treatment is with a variety of medications to slow the development of the bone changes and to reverse these changes to reduce symptoms.

Patients with Paget's disease who are asymptomatic are at little risk, although the deformities, such as enlargement of the skull or bowing of the legs, may be remarkably apparent. Your physician will advise you if you have bones that appear to be unusually susceptible to injury. Changes in the legs with bowing of the leg bones may cause some instability, and particular care should be taken to avoid falls.

Notify Our Office If

- You notice hats no longer fit your head.
- You notice you have become bowlegged.

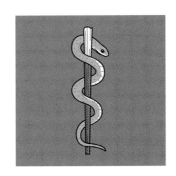
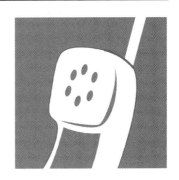

Fitness

Walking as Exercise

Patient and Caregiver's Guide

General Information

Walking is a form of activity that most of us engage in daily. In addition to being an activity of normal daily living, it is also a good form of exercise. It is best thought of as a low-intensity activity. It is generally safe, produces little injury, and is inexpensive. It suffers a bit from being such a natural and uncomplicated form of exercise that many doubt its benefits. There are significant benefits. Careful medical studies carried out over a decade have confirmed the health benefits of walking as exercise.

Generally, significant walkers (those who walk a mile or more daily) have half the mortality rate (measured as deaths per year) of individuals with only limited walking. The benefits seem to correlate best with the distance walked rather than the speed or effort expended in walking. There can be little question that walking is beneficial exercise.

Important Points in Application

Who can benefit from walking? Anyone except individuals who, perhaps, for medical reasons, have had to limit their exercise. There are a few individuals who, because of illness, have had their exercise limited and rest prescribed. Patients with heart failure often fall into that category. There are also some patients who must restrict walking because of potential damage to weight-bearing joints or because of inflammation in the legs. Patients with infections involving the joints or legs are examples. Most patients who can walk safely can exercise safely by walking. If you have any questions about the safety of walking as exercise, discuss them with your physician.

How much walking should you do? Real benefit occurs when you walk more than 1 mile. It is unwise to walk so far that you become fatigued and may have difficulty returning home. Often there is a period of conditioning or training necessary when beginning any kind of exercise, and you should not expect to walk long distances when first starting out. You should also remember that the distance walked seems more important than the speed at which you walk. By walking slowly, it is often possible to achieve your target distance without unnecessary fatigue. It is both reasonable and effective to split your daily walk into two or more shorter walks that together achieve your goal.

It is unwise to walk so far or so rapidly that it causes symptoms. When walking is suggested by your physician as part of the treatment for an underlying medical condition, it is best initiated under the direction of a therapist.

- Walk in a safe environment, preferably with someone else.
- Dress appropriately for the season and the weather.
- Select well-fitting shoes. Shoes designed for walking not only protect your feet but also help to prevent falls.

Notify Our Office If

- You wish to begin a program of walking as exercise but are concerned about the possible effects on your health.

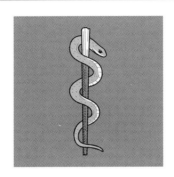
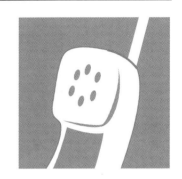

End of Life and Legal Issues

End of Life

Patient and Caregiver's Guide

General Information

Eventually, everyone dies. This is not a morbid thought, but rather a fact of life. Death may come as a result of accident or illness or may be the eventual result of the aging process.

Because the time of death, unlike the fact of death, is unpredictable, a prudent person should undertake some preparations for this eventuality. These preparations fall into two general areas: business and personal affairs and medical decisions, if one becomes incapacitated.

Business and personal affairs focus on the disposal of personal property and one's business relationships. Although these decisions are personal, there is often the need for help from financial counselors and attorneys to ensure that the wishes can be properly implemented. Seek professional help concerning the carrying out of your wishes.

The second general area involved in end-of-life planning concerns medical decisions. The concern is how and by whom your medical decisions will be made if you become incapacitated and unable to make these decisions for yourself.

There are four possible options for medical decision-making, if you become incapacitated. These are (1) guardianship, (2) living will, (3) durable power of attorney, and (4) next of kin. While you have capacity, you may select and change among some of these options. Remember that there is no way to avoid this issue. Not selecting any of the options means that you have, by default, selected the next of kin option. Two of these choices involve the use of a written legal document called an *advance directive*. The two remaining options depend on your kin or the courts to make the treatment decisions for you. If you have decided not to use an advance directive, then you have decided to permit your kin or the courts to act for you. You cannot waive making a decision.

Guardianship

Guardians are court-appointed individuals designated to act for you in business, personal, and health matters. They are usually appointed after incapacity occurs. At the court's option, the guardian may or may not be kin. Guardians are often appointed when kin disagree and cannot reach a decision.

Living Will

This is an advance directive document in which you can specify how you wish to be treated, if you become incapacitated. It is usually used to identify or to limit the use of life-sustaining treatments, such as resuscitation and artificial breathing supported by a machine. In some states, it may also be used to limit other forms of therapy.

A living will gives you autonomy over your health care decisions. The problem is that once you become mentally incapacitated, your instructions can no longer be modified to accommodate your changing health status. These changes may involve circumstances that you could not anticipate or predict.

Your physician can help you understand the meaning of your choices in light of your personal health history.

Durable Power of Attorney

This is an advance directive document in which you designate a person (surrogate) who will make your health-care decisions for you, if you become mentally incapacitated. You must choose an individual in whom you are willing to place your trust for life decisions and who is willing to accept that responsibility. It is wise and prudent to select an individual who understands your personal feelings concerning health care at the end of life so that he or she is able to interpret these wishes in the setting of your changing health care needs.

Next of Kin

If you do not elect to use an advance directive, then in the event of your incapacity, the laws of your state permit the decisions to be made by your next of kin. If the courts have intervened to appoint a guardian for you, the guardian will take precedence over your next of kin. If you are married, your spouse will be your next of kin. If you are single, widowed, or your spouse is incapacitated, other of your kin will be empowered to become your decision maker. Each state has an order of priority for which next of kin will be selected. Usually, this begins with your children, followed by parents, brothers and sisters, and more distant kin.

If you rely on next of kin, the choice of your decision maker will be left to chance and will depend on the circumstances, especially who can be contacted at the time of your incapacity.

 ## Notify Our Office If

- You wish to discuss any aspect of the use of an advance directive for health care decisions, if you become incapacitated.

Legal Issues

General Information

Each of us has the opportunity to control our own fate when faced with health-care issues. Remarkable advances in medical treatment can occasionally allow unwanted prolongation of medical attention. For patients who have clear wishes concerning their treatment in the event of serious debilitating illness, several options exist. These options include advance directives, living wills, and durable power of attorney.

Advance Directives

At the time of hospitalization, it is possible to designate that there are certain kinds of care that you do not wish to receive. Commonly, these are called DNR orders, meaning Do Not Resuscitate. This means that in the event of a sudden stopping of your heart or breathing, you have directed the physicians and other health care workers not to attempt to revive you. This type of order is often used when a patient has reached the end of an otherwise untreatable problem, such as terminal cancer.

The major drawback to this type of plan is the very terseness of the directive. It leaves the medical care personnel with a *yes* or *no* response in a *maybe* situation.

Living Wills

A living will is a more complete form of an advance directive. It is a written document containing an explanation of your preferences regarding intervention and life support. Preparation of a living will allows you, along with your physician, to include or exclude specific forms of care. It allows you to set conditions for the use of some treatments.

The drawback to living wills is that they become fixed at the time of signing. They can be revised as long as you are capable of changing them. During acute illnesses, circumstances change in ways that living wills cannot anticipate and at times when revision is not possible.

Durable Power of Attorney

Durable power of attorney permits a clear indication of your own preferences regarding various methods of life-saving care. It differs from a living will in that it also allows you to appoint a specific individual or individuals who, if you become incapacitated, will act for you. You give them your power of attorney. They know and understand your wishes but are also able to interpret them in light of changing circumstances.

The principal problem may be the selection of a person to act for you (your surrogate). Also, if you do not select a surrogate, decisions may be made for you by an available next of kin, not necessarily by the person you might select.

Implementation

The options available regarding health-care choices differ by state. Your physician will know or will direct you to someone familiar with the options available to you. Seek the counsel of your family and your physician to understand fully what possible care you are selecting and what you are excluding.

 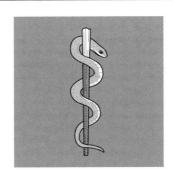 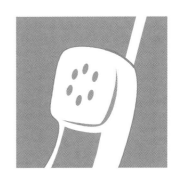

Charts and Diagrams

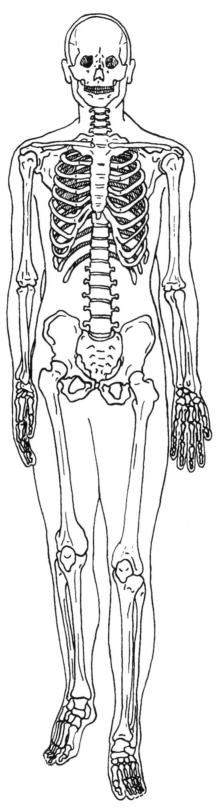

The skeletal system, showing major bones and joints. (From Griffith HW. Instructions for Patients, 5th ed. Philadelphia, WB Saunders, 1994, p 591.)

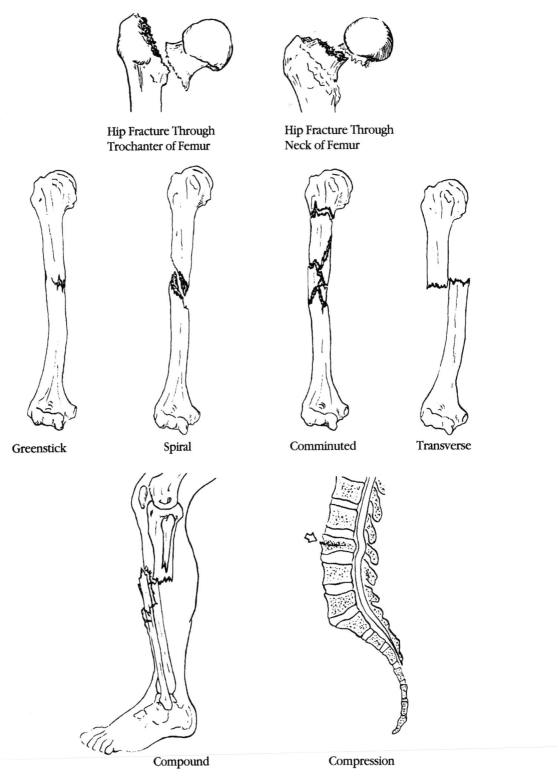

Hip Fracture Through
Trochanter of Femur

Hip Fracture Through
Neck of Femur

Greenstick

Spiral

Comminuted

Transverse

Compound

Compression

Types of fractures. (From Griffith HW. Instructions for Patients, 5th ed. Philadelphia, WB Saunders, 1994, p 592.)

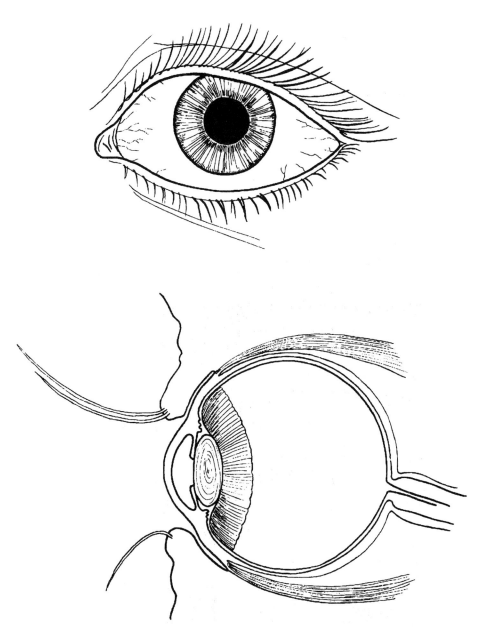

The eye. (From Griffith HW. Instructions for Patients, 5th ed. Philadelphia, WB Saunders, 1994, p 576.)

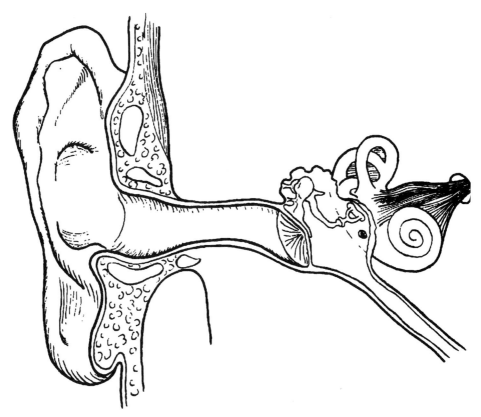

The ear. (From Griffith HW. Instructions for Patients, 5th ed. Philadelphia, WB Saunders, 1994, p 577.)

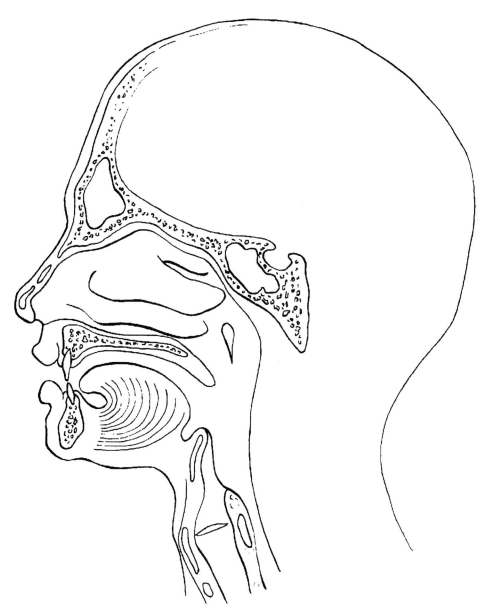

The nose and throat. (From Griffith HW. Instructions for Patients, 5th ed. Philadelphia, WB Saunders, 1994, p 578.)

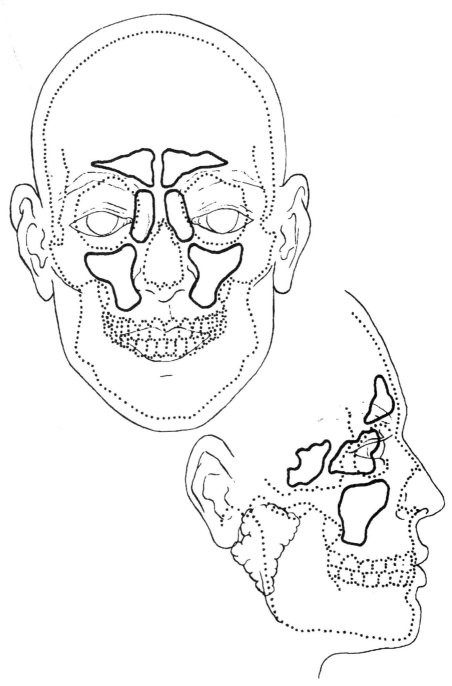

The sinus cavities. (From Griffith HW. Instructions for Patients, 5th ed. Philadelphia, WB Saunders, 1994, p 579.)

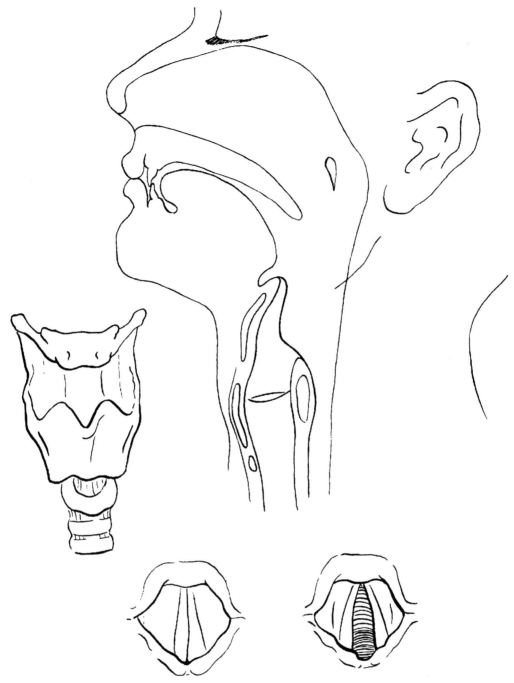

The trachea and larynx. (From Griffith HW. Instructions for Patients, 5th ed. Philadelphia, WB Saunders, 1994, p 580.)

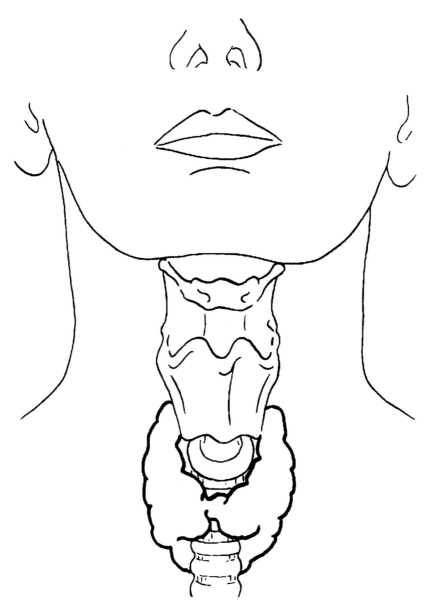

The larynx and thyroid gland. (From Griffith HW. Instructions for Patients, 5th ed. Philadelphia, WB Saunders, 1994, p 581.)

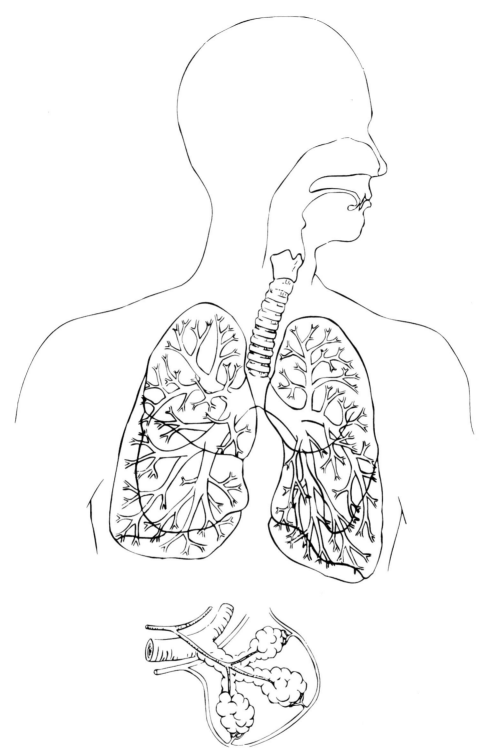

The bronchial tree and lungs. (From Griffith HW. Instructions for Patients, 5th ed. Philadelphia, WB Saunders, 1994, p 582.)

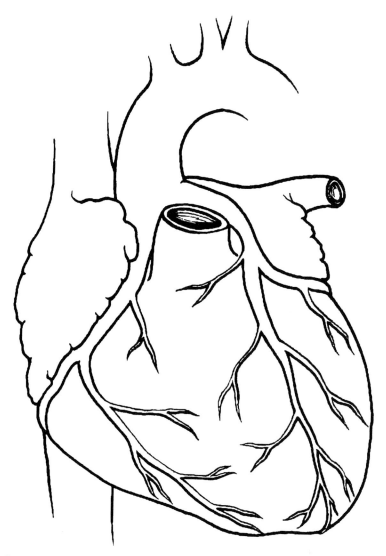

The heart, showing the coronary arteries. (From Griffith HW. Instructions for Patients, 5th ed. Philadelphia, WB Saunders, 1994, p 583.)

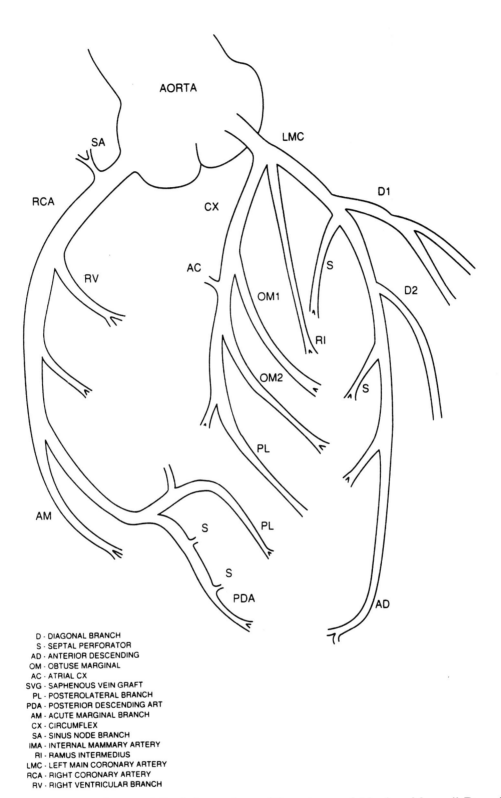

AORTA

SA

LMC

RCA

CX

D1

RV

AC

S

OM1

D2

RI

OM2

S

PL

AM

S

PL

S

PDA

AD

D - DIAGONAL BRANCH
S - SEPTAL PERFORATOR
AD - ANTERIOR DESCENDING
OM - OBTUSE MARGINAL
AC - ATRIAL CX
SVG - SAPHENOUS VEIN GRAFT
PL - POSTEROLATERAL BRANCH
PDA - POSTERIOR DESCENDING ART
AM - ACUTE MARGINAL BRANCH
CX - CIRCUMFLEX
SA - SINUS NODE BRANCH
IMA - INTERNAL MAMMARY ARTERY
RI - RAMUS INTERMEDIUS
LMC - LEFT MAIN CORONARY ARTERY
RCA - RIGHT CORONARY ARTERY
RV - RIGHT VENTRICULAR BRANCH

The coronary arteries and their branches. (Courtesy of Marion Merrell Dow Inc., Kansas City, MO.)

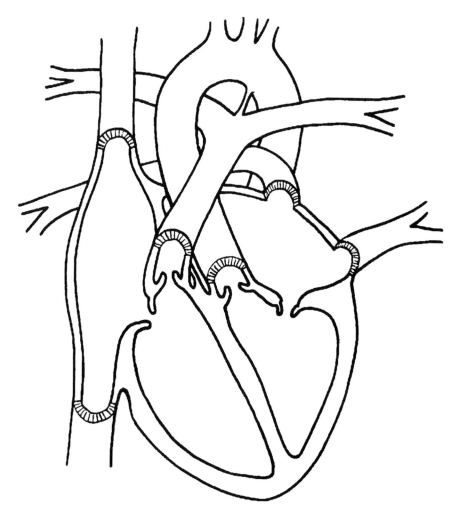

The heart, schematic cross section. (From Griffith HW. Instructions for Patients, 5th ed. Philadelphia, WB Saunders, 1994, p 584.)

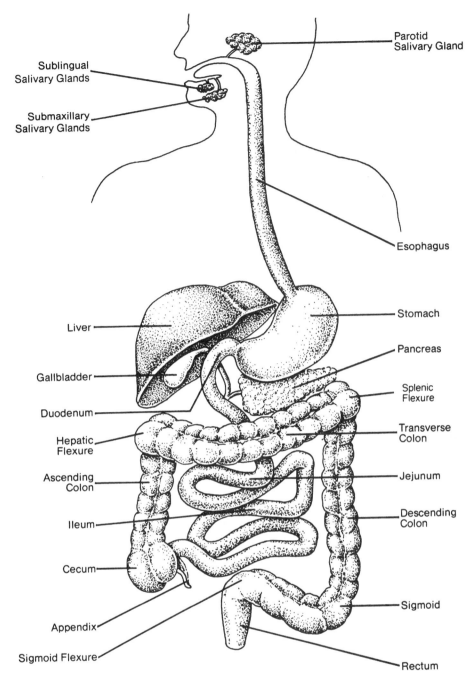

The digestive system. (Courtesy of Crohn's and Colitis Foundation of America, Inc., New York.)

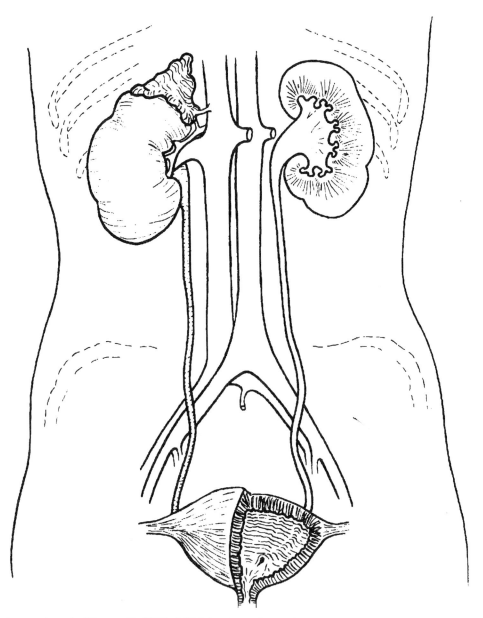

The urinary tract. (From Griffith HW. Instructions for Patients, 5th ed. Philadelphia, WB Saunders, 1994, p 587.)

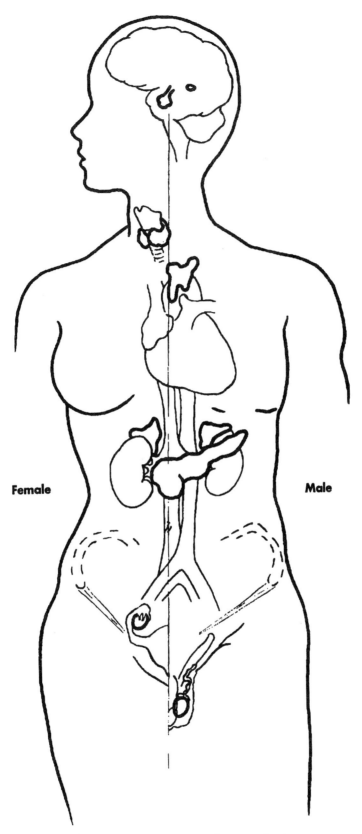

Female

Male

The endocrine system, female and male. (From Griffith HW. Instructions for Patients, 5th ed. Philadelphia, WB Saunders, 1994, p 588.)

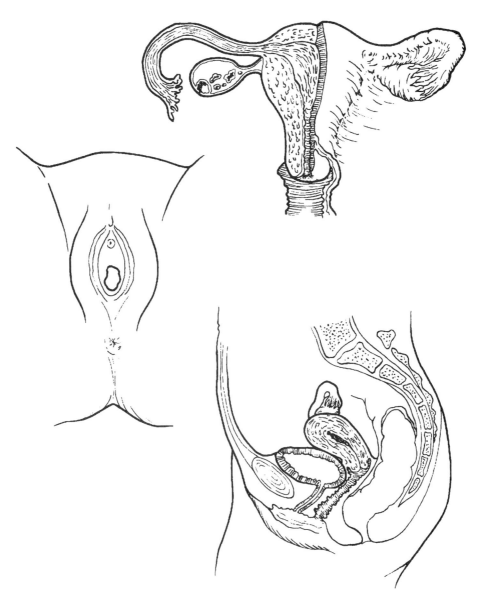

The female genital organs. (From Griffith HW. Instructions for Patients, 5th ed. Philadelphia, WB Saunders, 1994, p 589.)

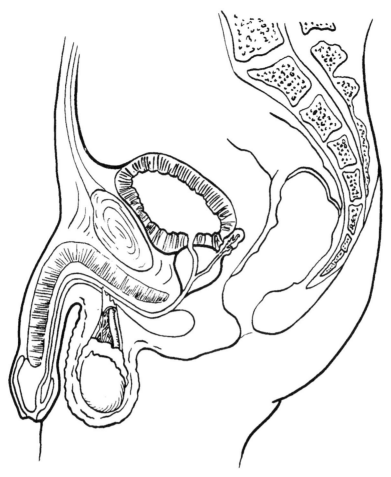

The male genital organs. (From Griffith HW. Instructions for Patients, 5th ed. Philadelphia, WB Saunders, 1994, p 590.)